The Body
and Health

Brian Ward

Macdonald Guidelines

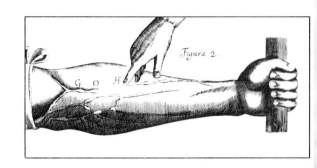

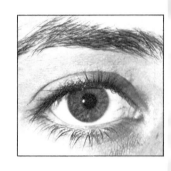

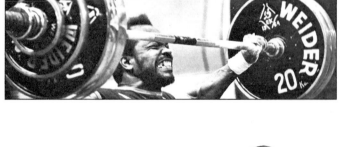

Editorial Manager
Chester Fisher
Series editor
Jim Miles
Designer
Peter Benoist
Picture research
Frances Middlestorb
Production
Philip Hughes

ISBN 0 356 06003 9

© Macdonald Educational Ltd 1976

First published 1976
Reprinted 1978
Macdonald Educational Ltd,
Holywell House, Worship Street,
London EC2A 2EN

Made and printed by
Waterlow (Dunstable) Limited

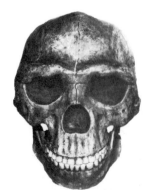

Contents

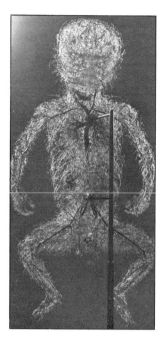

Information
4   Introducing the body; a complex machine
6   Evolution; our family tree
10 The tribes of man
12 Biorhythms; what makes us tick?
16 The human frame; strength of purpose
20 Muscles; a team of motors
24 Blood; ten pints of life
28 The vital organs; the body's powerhouse
34 The nervous system; our personal
        messengers
37 The brain; imagination and control
42 Sensing the world; the five wonders
46 Skin; not just a pretty wrapper
48 The digestive system; fuel and how
        we burn it
52 Glands; preparing for action
55 Reproducing mankind; more than
        multiplication
60 Age and ageing; the inescapable conclusion

Activities
62 First aid; artificial respiration
64 Self treatment
66 Looking after your body
68 Exercising care
72 Can you trust your senses?
74 How emotional are you?

Reference
76 Eating the right way
78 Nutrition; tables of needs
80 Food of nations
81 Life expectancy; causes of death
82 The skeleton
83 The muscles
84 Blood circulation
85 The vital organs
86 The nervous system
87 Height/weight chart
88 Book list
90 General information
91 Glossary
93 Index

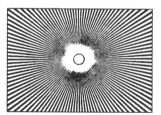

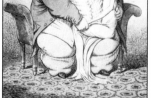

Introducing the body

Mankind is an animal which has never quite grown up. Measured against other mammals, man is remarkably like an overgrown embryo. We have large heads, comparatively small limbs, and a skin texture like that of most new-born mammals. Our finger and toenails are poor substitutes for those of other creatures, and we do not even have a properly developed protective coat, making do with odd patches of hair about our heads, faces, and bodies.

The live computer

What really makes us unique, and compensates for our physical deficiencies, is the human brain. Over the last 100,000 years we have developed a brain which makes man the dominant species on our planet. Our brain differs physically from those of our nearest relatives, the apes, largely in its greater size. But having a bigger brain does not simply make us extra-clever apes. It allows us, alone among all known life, to create abstract concepts, to have a sense of humour, and above all, to possess language.

The gift of communication gives us our humanity. We can pass complex ideas from one person to the next, and having invented language, can pass on the accumulated learning of one generation to the next, ensuring that our total body of knowledge is steadily increased.

Our smallest parts

We share basic physical structures in common with other mammals. Our bodies are built up from millions of cells, which are grouped together to form tissues and organs, each with a particular function. The skin which covers most of our external surface is a complex organ which protects the delicate tissues beneath. But at the same time it acts as a radiator to cool the body, or as an insulator to prevent too much loss of heat.

Although the skin is built up from living cells, the ones we see are dead, and in the process of being sloughed off.

Beneath the skin, we have a number of quite distinct groups of structures. The skeleton is the basic framework on which we are built. It serves to support us, and to protect the most crucial organs of the body, forming a rigid box about the brain, our most important single organ. The ribs and spine make a flexible armour around most of the internal organs.

Human motors

The muscles form another major group of structures. They work with the skeleton to move the body and implement the commands of the brain. The internal organs themselves provide the motor for the human machine. They enable us to fuel our bodies with easily available material; the air we breathe and the food we eat. They pump this fuel around the body through many miles of blood vessels which range down to microscopic size. They also extract impurities from the blood, as the waste products accumulate, and dispose of them outside the body.

The whole system operates like a miniaturised self-repairing factory, controlled by a brain which is thousands of times more efficient than the best computer mankind has ever built.

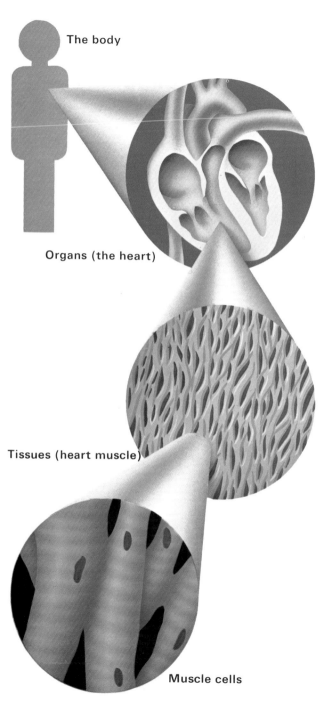

The body

Organs (the heart)

Tissues (heart muscle)

Muscle cells

The body and its vital organs are made up from a number of simple units — the cells. From these simple building-blocks, tissues are constructed, consisting of huge numbers of cells grouped together to perform a specific task. In turn, tissues are built into organs, which consist of a complex assembly of different types of tissue, each with its own special function. Individual cells are minute, and are too small to be seen with the naked eye. They vary enormously in shape and function. The simplest cell of all is found in connective tissue, and is a shapeless blob of life, whose function is to fill apertures between other types of cell or tissues. At the opposite extreme is the nerve cell, which is extremely specialised for its task of conveying messages through the body. Although it is still minute, the nerve cell bears a fibre which can be as much as 1.5 m (5ft) in length. In both connective tissue and nerve tissue, the cells are bunched together by the million, forming parts of even more complex organ systems. Heart muscle is a good example of this build-up of tissues. An individual cell is a threadlike object, which even in isolation will contract regularly. But built into a web of tissue, somehow all the cells manage to contract simultaneously.

Evolution

Even towards the end of the 20th century, the problem of the origins of man are far from settled. To many people, the idea that we are "descended from monkeys" is distasteful, and this view has been aired ever since Charles Darwin first published his theories on evolution. The facts are somewhat different; mankind, and all surviving apes and monkeys, are descendents of a common ancestor. The modern chimpanzee resembles this common ancestor no more than do we ourselves.

Special features

What are the features which make man so different from other animals? Our brain is obviously far superior to that of other animals, and it is this which allows us to be the dominant form of life on this planet. But we have a number of physical peculiarities, none of which are exclusive to man, but in combination give us the physical abilities to complement our astonishing brains. Mankind and his closest relatives are characterised by:

1 A very flexible system of limbs, not specialised for any particular function.
2 Very mobile fingers.
3 Nails to help us grip, rather than claws.
4 A shortened nose, with a corresponding loss of the power to smell.
5 Good eyesight, with binocular vision, resulting from the placing of eyes at the front of the head.
6 Teeth which can cope with almost any diet, either vegetable, or meat.
7 A very small number of offspring at each pregnancy, a protracted pregnancy, and a very long period of care for the offspring.

Biologically speaking, mankind is an

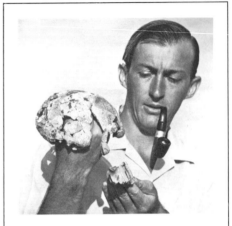

In 1972, Richard Leakey discovered the remains of the first man known to have made and used tools. On the shores of Lake Rudolf, in Northern Kenya, Leakey found deliberately chipped flints which could have been used for hunting small game, and for skinning the catch. They were made by a "man" about 1.5 m tall, and with a brain twice the size of a chimpanzee's. He lived 2 million years ago.

infant. We have walked the earth, as recognisable men, for a mere 2 million years or so. And the primitive men who developed cave paintings appeared only 2,000 generations ago. This may seem a vast span of time, but pales into insignificance when seen against the earth's geological history. The dinosaurs were the dominant form of life for 155 million years, and even today's reptiles are still similar to their ancestors of 300 million years ago.

The broken chain

We know in great detail how mammals like horses developed. An almost unbroken chain of fossils exists, showing their slow evolution from small rodent-like animals to the horses we know today. But all the known fossils of man's ancestors could be fitted into a couple of suitcases—about 1,500 fragments of bones and teeth. Nowhere was primitive man common enough to leave more than a few traces, and these are not enough to provide a complete record.

However, the course of our evolution is fairly clear, although the dating of some remains is doubtful and mankind may have emerged much earlier than was formerly thought.

It is thought that we ultimately descend from a shrew-like animal, similar to the tree shrews still surviving in Malaysia and Indonesia. From these came monkey-like creatures, which in turn gave rise to monkeys, apes, and our own predecessors. Some paleontologists believe that the final development of man took place in Africa, where many recent fossil finds have been made. Here in the Olduvai Gorge in Tanzania, and by nearby Lake Rudolf, the remains of Homo habilis have been identified; a true man about 1.2 m high, with a brain half the size of ours, and a man-like hand, who lived about $2\frac{1}{2}$ million years ago.

Merging and emerging

Because evolution is a process of continuous slow change, one species merging imperceptibly into another, it is seldom possible to identify the fragmentary remains with any certainty. Older fossils, called Australopithecus, are much closer to apes than to man. Moving forward to more obviously human creatures, yet another type, Homo erectus, appeared around a million years ago, and his remains have been found throughout the Far East. Then one branch of man took an evolutionary blind alley, resulting in Neanderthal man; a heavily-built race with bulging jaw, receding forehead, and protruding ridges over the eyes. He was not one of our direct ancestors, and soon disappeared, perhaps pushed out by emerging modern man, Homo sapiens. Oddly enough, the brain of the Neanderthal was bigger than our own, but this did not ensure his survival.

Even the emergence of man in a form physically identical with our own did not immediately give us mastery of the earth. It was many thousands of years before we began the population explosion which ensured our dominance.

▼ Externally the dolphin looks like a fish, but its skeleton gives away its relationship to man. The "hands" are almost identical in structure.

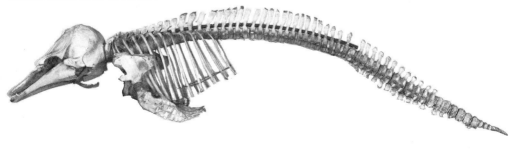

The appearance of man

When did man first emerge from his ape-like ancestors? Half-a-million years ago, most authorities would have said, until very recently. But now, almost every year fossils are unearthed in Africa which push back the origins of man by millions of years. It seems that the earliest types of true man appeared 2½ million years ago or more. Man did not suddenly emerge from apes, and among the sparse fossil records are a number of remains which could be either ape-man or man-like ape. Primitive man was never common, and our ape ancestors were even rarer, so it is difficult to produce an unbroken family tree for mankind.

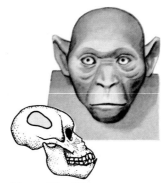

About 25 millions years ago lived an ape called Proconsul. This may be the earliest of our direct ancestors, as it had a number of potentially man-like features to its skeleton.

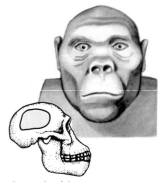

Australopithecus was a man-like ape which lived in Africa about 5 million years ago. It was probably not our direct ancestor, but had a number of man-like features, and used primitive tools.

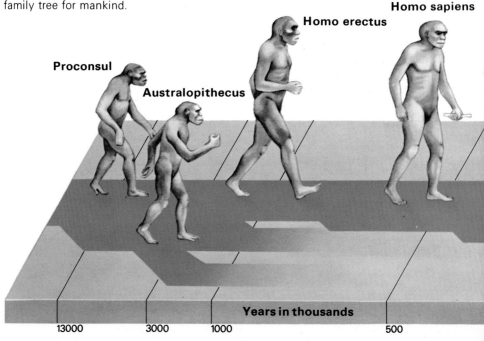

Proconsul

Australopithecus

Homo erectus

Homo sapiens

Years in thousands

13000   3000   1000   500

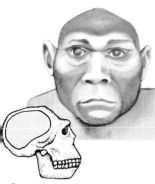

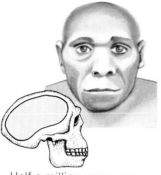

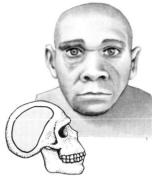

One of the earliest known true men was Homo erectus, living in Java a million years ago. His brain was quite large, and he made flint tools, and understood the use of fire.

Half a million years ago Homo erectus still thrived, living in caves near Pekin. His brain was now much larger, and his skull was losing the ape-like jaw and heavy eyebrows of Java man.

70,000 years ago, in Europe, Neanderthal man appeared. He was a heavily-built, brutish-looking creature, who resembled his earlier ancestors. He was pushed out by emergent modern man.

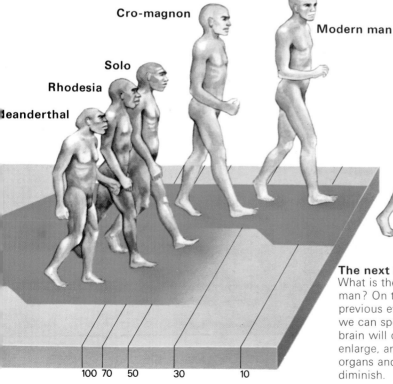

Cro-magnon

Modern man

Solo

Rhodesia

Neanderthal

100 70 50   30   10

The next step?
What is the future for man? On the basis of our previous evolutionary past, we can speculate that our brain will continue to enlarge, and unwanted organs and appendages diminish.

The tribes of man

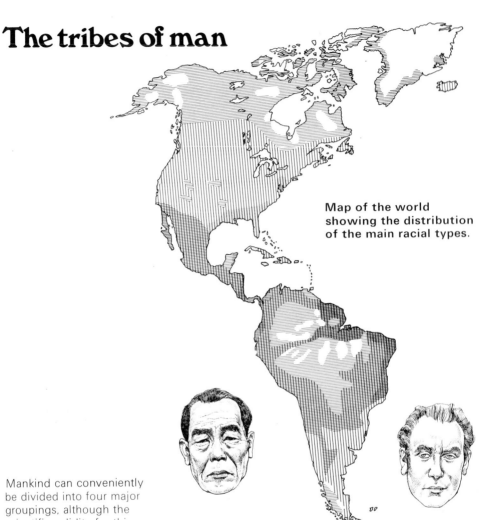

Map of the world
showing the distribution
of the main racial types.

Mankind can conveniently
be divided into four major
groupings, although the
scientific validity for this
subdivision is doubtful.
We are all of a single
species, in spite of the
tremendous variation
between the different
races. The biological test
of a species is that its
members must be able to
interbreed, and of course,
even the most diverse
races of man can and do
intermarry and produce
children.

Mongoloids comprise the
asiatic races, with slanted
eyes, yellowish skin, and
straight black hair. This
grouping can be stretched
to allow the inclusion of
North and South American
Indians, with their reddish
skins, and Eskimos who
are distributed around the
Arctic circle. This group
comprises a third of the
human race.

The Caucasoids or "white"
races are by far the most
plentiful. Caucasoids
include not only the
European types, but also
Indians, Arabs, and Jews.
They can vary from the
fair-skinned European to
the nearly-black inhabitants
of Bengal, but have
uniformly thin faces and
straight hair.

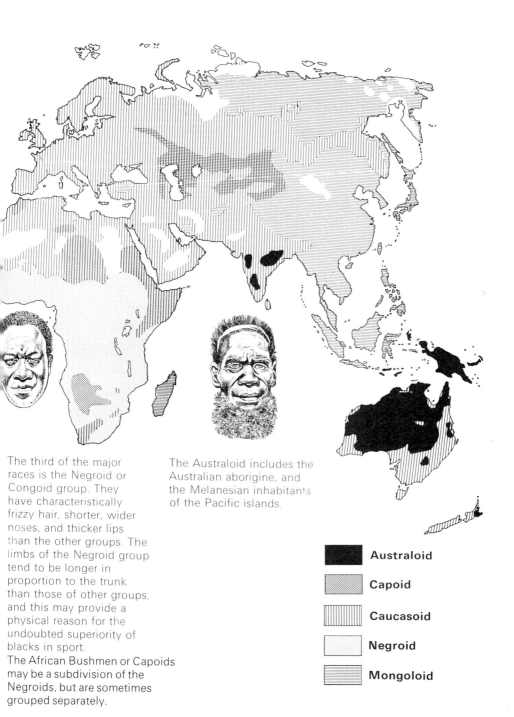

The third of the major races is the Negroid or Congoid group. They have characteristically frizzy hair, shorter, wider noses, and thicker lips than the other groups. The limbs of the Negroid group tend to be longer in proportion to the trunk than those of other groups, and this may provide a physical reason for the undoubted superiority of blacks in sport.
The African Bushmen or Capoids may be a subdivision of the Negroids, but are sometimes grouped separately.

The Australoid includes the Australian aborigine, and the Melanesian inhabitants of the Pacific islands.

- Australoid
- Capoid
- Caucasoid
- Negroid
- Mongoloid

Biorhythms

Through our bodies courses a continually fluctuating tide of chemicals. The amounts in our bloodstream vary from hour to hour; day to day; and as we age, vary over the years. In a healthy body, they vary in strictly determined sequence, producing recurring cycles, or biorhythms.

Minute quantities of chemical substances can have dramatic effects on behaviour. These may be hormones (chemical messengers) or even the normal nutrients present in the blood. As these substances ebb and flow in strict rotation, they produce regular cycles of behaviour, by which we time our daily activities.

The 25 hour day

The most obvious human biological rhythm is sleep, which normally occupies the same spot in our 24-hour living cycle. We usually assume that the "correct" time for sleep is controlled by daylight, and that it is "natural" to sleep at night. But if a person is completely shut off from contact with the outside world for several weeks in a deep cave, without a clock, his body still follows the normal cycle of sleeping and wakefulness. The only difference is that he generally follows a 25-hour day under these free-running conditions.

So our daily cycle, or circadian rhythm, is locked in the complexities of our bodies, and daylight and darkness, or the use of clocks, simply correct any minor discrepancies in our 24-hour cycle. This overriding control can be easily disturbed, however, during long distance east/west flights into different time zones, when various of the body's rhythms become hopelessly confused and out of sequence. The end result is jet-lag—several days of tiredness, confusion, headaches, and insomnia, which can cause problems for those who travel a great deal.

Rhythms of resistance

The periodic tides of chemicals which ebb and flow in our bloodstreams can have great importance in maintaining health, and in fighting disease. Susceptibility to infection or to poisons varies widely at different times in the circadian cycle. Animal experiments have shown that a

---

We are all built around an accurate biological clock, yet many of us have a very poor sense of time. Some people are able to sit down in an armchair for a 20-minute nap, and will wake up within a few minutes of the time they set themselves—others would sleep on for many hours. How do they known when to wake? Our body physiology clearly has a good time sense, telling us when to eat, and changing the chemical constituents of the blood regularly, at the same time of day or night. When there are no outside cues, like clocks or daylight, we are forced to rely on our internal clocks. Even a man buried hundreds of feet underground in a cave continues his regular rhythms of sleeping and waking, although they are no longer exactly based on a 12-hour cycle. Gradually his time sense will become more and more distorted.

1 Brain activity
2 Skin growth
3 Urine; rate of excretion
4 Plasma: protein in blood
5 Body temperature (oral)
6 Body; physical vigour
7 Body weight
8 Heart rate
9 Blood pressure; systolic

10 Blood pressure; diastolic
11 Expiratory peak flow
12 Respiratory rate
13 Skin; allergy to house dust
14 Skin; allergy to grass pollen
15 Tooth pain
16 Birth—spontaneous
17 Death from surgery
18 Death from air accidents
19 Miscellaneous deaths

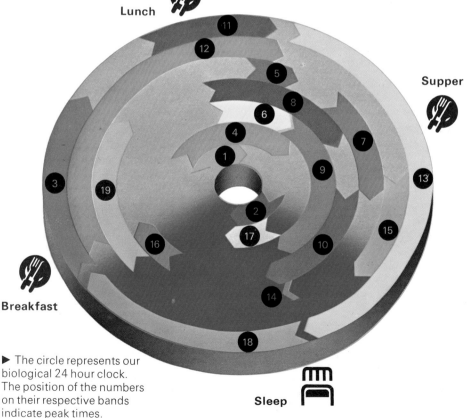

Lunch

Supper

Breakfast

Sleep

▶ The circle represents our biological 24 hour clock. The position of the numbers on their respective bands indicate peak times.

dose of bacteria or chemicals which normally kill a rat may not prove fatal if given at a different time of day. This has a number of serious implications for medical science, which are now being closely studied. Powerful drugs may prove toxic if taken at the wrong part of the biological cycle. Equally, there may be a best time of day to take a drug to ensure maximum benefit.

Illnesses like epilepsy seem to be closely tied in to the circadian rhythm, and researchers have found that epileptic seizures tend to occur in the mornings. Even pain seems more acute at certain times of day. Hospitals find that patients request painkillers much more frequently in the night than during the daylight hours. Is this because pain preys more on the mind in the dark and loneliness of a ward? Some researchers have associated this increased susceptibility with increased levels of hormones in the blood, liberated by the adrenal glands.

The key to body time is probably built into the cell, as when organs, or even individual cells, are separated from the body, they continue to function in their circadian rhythms. This is not a prerogative of higher animals, as primitive organisms and even plants show similar cycles of activity. But the precise mechanism remains a mystery.

Our ups and downs

The effects of our circadian rhythm, and of slower rhythms like a woman's menstrual cycle, have profound influence on mood, concentration, and behaviour. We all acknowledge a time of day when we reach a mental peak, whether morning, afternoon, or evening, and this peak varies between individuals. But with most people, the senses are at a peak in late evening, and in the small hours. This is why sounds seem so loud when we are trying to get back to sleep.

▼ The word "lunatic" reflects the ancient belief that madness was influenced by the moon. Asylums were filled with people whose problems often made them objects of derision.

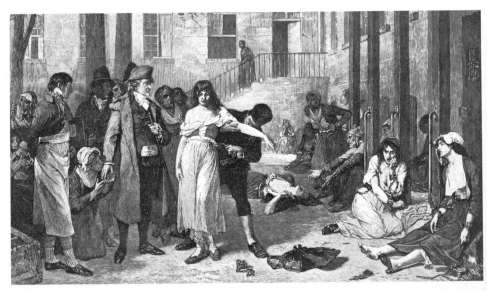

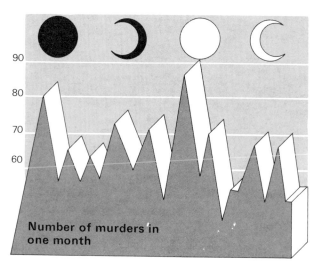

90

80

70

60

Number of murders in one month

◀ By studying statistics on murders committed between 1956–1970, in Florida, psychiatrists found a close relationship between violent crime and the phases of the moon. Particularly violent murders rose to a peak at new moon, and again at full moon. The same tendency was found in other areas of the U.S.A., but so far, no logical explanation has been found.

The causes of these mental changes are not understood, but may perhaps be related to circadian rhythms in the proportions of the tiny traces of chemicals which relay signals in the nervous system.

Biological lunacy

The monthly rhythm is deeply ingrained in us. Menstruation follows an approximately monthly cycle, but even in males, a monthly rhythm can be detected in hormones circulating in the bloodstream, although the effects this has on behaviour is not clear. It is now obvious, however, that the ancient superstition that madness was brought on by the phases of the moon contains more than a germ of truth. Study of the records of large mental hospitals frequently shows that disturbances among patients recur at about monthly intervals, though not necessarily at full moon.

This may be because in a group of people biorhythms have a tendency to become synchronised. People following the same daily, weekly, and monthly routines gradually edge their biorhythms towards a common cycle, where all sleep and eat at the same time.

Getting the rhythm

Some quite serious mental diseases follow a rhythmic pattern, such as manic-depression, when periods of excitement are followed by deep melancholy. This cycle can alternate over periods as short as 48 hours, or over several years. Even the common mild depressive illnesses can recurr in this way, although the period between these episodes is usually so long that no rhythm is apparent.

In many cases of mental disturbance, it has been found that the normal sequence of biorhythms is upset. When the delicate chemical balance within the body is affected, and hormones are poured into the blood in unaccustomed proportions, it is not surprising that mental and physical disturbances follow. Biorhythms are a new and controversial area of research, and no new methods of treatment based on the study of biorhythms have yet been perfected.

The human frame

Many millions of years ago, a primitive form of life stepped aside from the line of evolution, and developed internal strengthening which gave rise to animals with backbones, culminating in man. In many primitive animals, an external shell or jointed armour forms a protection against enemies. It also provides a solid base against which muscles can pull when the animal moves. But it has a severe drawback —the growth rate and maximum size of the animal is severely restricted.

Vertebrates have overcome this problem by developing an *internal* skeleton, which grows at the same rate as other tissues. The skeleton supports the body, and allows rapid movement when necessary. At the same time, the most vulnerable parts of the body continue to be well protected.

Versatile protection

The skull surrounds the brain—our most crucial organ. The whole structure around the brain is nearly spherical—and in engineering terms, a hollow sphere is one of the strongest known structures.

The spinal cord is almost as important as the brain, and is encased in vertebrae. These are a series of bony rings, jointed together in such a way that they allow bending of the whole spinal column without damaging the delicate cord within. At the same time, the spine possesses enough "springiness" to return to its erect position, due to the cushioning discs of resilient cartilage between each vertebra.

▶Photomicrograph of a bone cell.

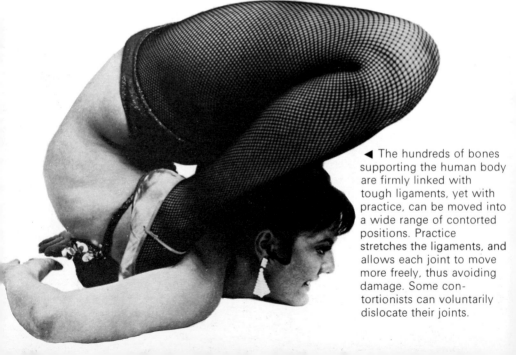

◀ The hundreds of bones supporting the human body are firmly linked with tough ligaments, yet with practice, can be moved into a wide range of contorted positions. Practice stretches the ligaments, and allows each joint to move more freely, thus avoiding damage. Some contortionists can voluntarily dislocate their joints.

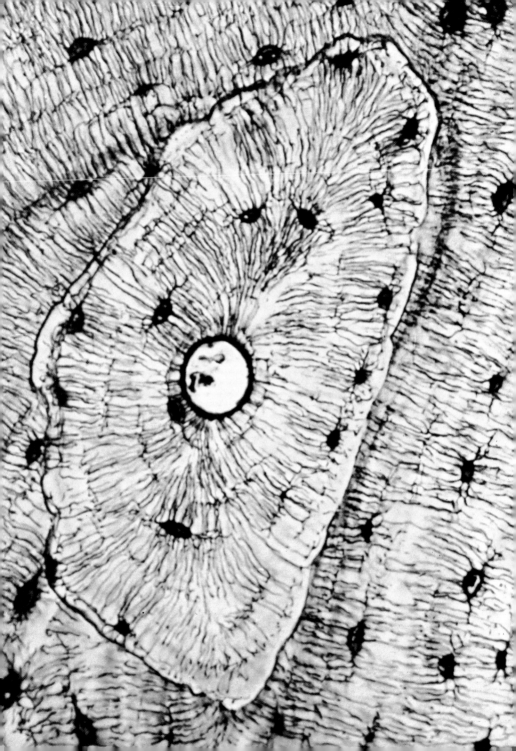

Joints are necessary wherever bones touch. Sometimes they are fixed rigidly, as in the bones of the skull, but more often they are hinged to allow movement in various directions. Joints allow the bones to hinge or rotate often under considerable load, yet they must be durable enough to last for a life-time. In some cases, like the spine (**6**), the joints which permit movement also impart rigidity to the structure by limiting the amount of movement possible.

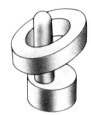

A special pivot joint (**1**) is needed where the skull meets the spine, to allow the head to rotate and to rock back and forth. A peg on the axis vertebra fits into a bony ring on the atlas vertebra.

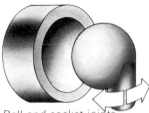

Ball and socket joints articulate the hip and the shoulder (**2**). The head of the bone fits tightly into a cartilage-lined cup, allowing rotation.

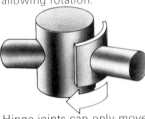

Hinge joints can only move in one direction (**3**). They are found in fingers and toes, ankles, and the elbows.

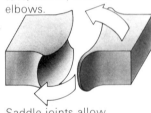

Saddle joints allow movement in two directions, while preventing rotation (**4**). The thumb has a saddle joint.

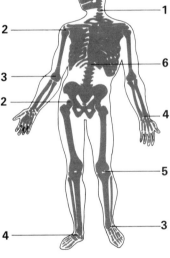

The knee joint (**5**) is subjected to tremendous strains, and is stabilised by ligaments which cross over inside the joint.

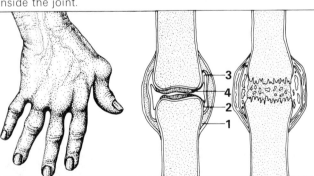

Many joints contain a synovial capsule (**1**); a fluid-filled bag (**2**), surrounded by tough membranes (**3**), allowing movement while preventing excess wear on the rubbery cartilage (**4**). In arthritis, this mechanism is destroyed and the bones become immobile.

Other bones have similar functions. The ribs, for example, surround the lungs and heart with a springy cage which both protects the organs, and assists with breathing. The pelvis, or hip bone, provides a firm base on which the legs articulate, and at the same time, forms a protective shield about the delicate organs of the abdomen.

Living rock

Altogether, adults have 106 bones in their bodies, although a new-born child may have more than 300. Several of these bones fuse together during development, however, producing a much smaller number at adulthood.

Bones are living tissues, and consist of layers of cells surrounded by hard layers of calcium phosphate and other minerals, looking rather like an onion in cross-section. The thigh bone is the strongest bone in the body, and daily withstands a pressure of 84 kg/cm^2 (1,200 lb/in^2) when an average size person walks normally and up to 300 kg/cm^2 (2 tons/in^2) during exertion.

The key to the light yet strong structure of bones is that they are usually hollow. In a tubular structure, most of the stresses and strains take place at the surface, so bones normally have a hard exterior, and a spongy central core.

In a new-born child, the skeleton is composed of rubbery cartilage, and the skull and limbs are quite flexible. As the child grows, harder tissues develop, starting in the middle of the long bones of the limbs, and gradually spreading along the shafts. As this tissue is laid down, the bones increase in thickness and in length, until by the age of 25, all growth ceases.

Repairing bone

Bone has a remarkable capacity to heal itself, although normal bone growth may long have ceased. Within a few days of fracturing a bone, minerals from the damaged ends are re-absorbed by the blood stream. The tissue remaining is soft, like that of a child. Fibrous tissues grow around the fracture, holding the broken section together, and within this fibrous mass, fresh calcium is deposited. After a few weeks, bone is produced about the damaged area, and a thickened strengthening area may be formed to reinforce the damaged part.

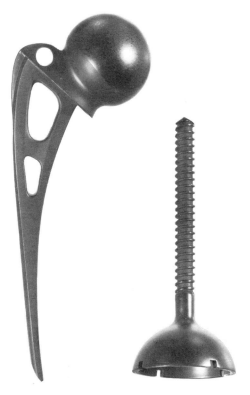

▼ Modern surgical techniques and newly developed materials allow many of the major joints of the body to be replaced. Shown below are the components of an artificial hip joint made from extremely durable material.

Muscles

Every movement we make results from muscular activity. From blinking the eye to kicking a ball, muscles are in action. Many of the activities of our internal organs are also controlled by muscles, although we are not usually aware of their operation. These two distinct types of muscle are called *voluntary* and *involuntary* muscle, and both are controlled by the nervous system.

Voluntary muscles

Voluntary muscles are under our direct control, and are responsible for all our normal daily activities. They make up the bulk of our flesh; about half of the body by weight. Viewed under the microscope, voluntary muscle can be seen to consist of bundles of tiny fibres running parallel to each other. Each of these fibres is capable of contracting when it receives the appropriate signal from the nervous system. Voluntary muscles are generally attached to a tough rope-like tendon, which is in turn firmly fixed to a ridge of bone. As the muscle contracts, it pulls on the tendon and causes the bone to move, flexed about its joint.

Many muscles are paired; one muscle may flex a limb, then the other straightens it. Sometimes a muscle moves other types of tissue. Facial muscles, for example, have one end attached to the bone of the skull, while the other end terminates in the tissues just beneath the skin. Laughter, tension, sadness, or anger are all portrayed on our faces by the action of the underlying

▶ Competitive sport places the body under strains for which it was never designed. Training develops a very high degree of speed and coordination for which Rod Laver is famous. The continual use of his left arm has developed it quite visibly.

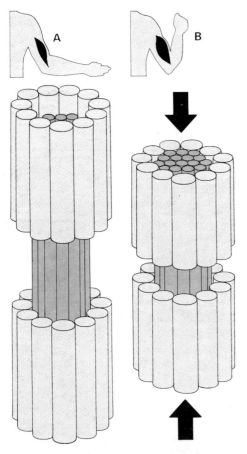

◀ Muscle tissue is built up from bundles of fibres, which contract in response to a signal from the nervous system. These bundles are packed into groups which make up a complete muscle. Illustration **A** shows the muscle in a relaxed state and **B** when it has contracted.

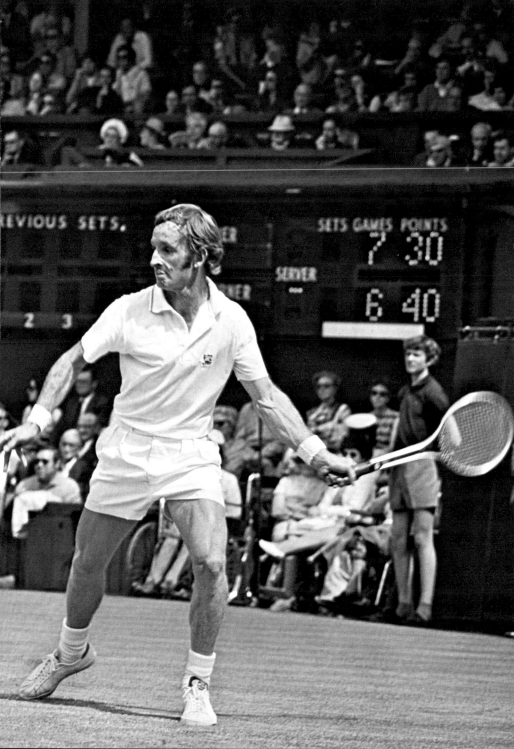

muscles.

The development of voluntary muscle depends largely on the amount of use it receives. "Muscle-building" exercises are aptly named, for muscle tissue increases in response to demand. Equally, however, it will diminish when not required, as can be seen when a broken limb is immobilised with plaster for a prolonged length of time. This wasting of unused muscle tissue is even more apparent when limbs are not used at all, as when a person is paralysed.

Involuntary muscles

Involuntary muscles operate the systems

▼ When relaxed in sleep, the human face is expressionless. Emotions are conveyed by varying the tension in the complex sets of muscles underlying the face, and are epitomised by the art of mime. Marcel Marceau is a great exponent of this art. He is able to master his body and facial muscles to create many varied illusions.

controlling our bodies. The heart is largely composed of a particular type of involuntary muscle, which contracts and relaxes regularly for our entire life. This regular heartbeat is largely automatic, and will continue even if the heart is surgically severed from the nervous system. Its speed and intensity of contraction, however, are controlled by the nervous system and hormones circulating in the blood, which cause it to work harder during violent exercise and at times of stress.

Other types of involuntary muscle are found in the walls of the intestine, where they produce wave-like contractions called peristalsis, which move the food along. Involuntary muscle is also found in the walls of arteries and in the bladder.

Feeding muscles

Muscles need energy when they contract, and this is obtained from glucose in the blood. After fierce muscular exertion, waste products from this process build up in the muscle tissues in the form of lactic

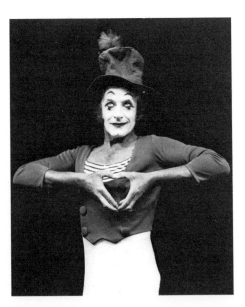

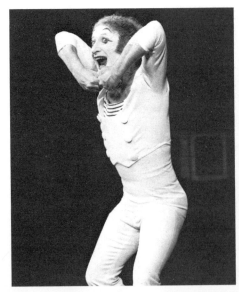

acid, reducing the efficiency of the muscle, and causing it to tire. Extra oxygen is needed to remove lactic acid from the system, so we breathe more deeply after exertion. Muscles involved in continual activity require large quantities of food and oxygen, so they have a plentiful blood supply.

Muscle tone

Normally, muscles are kept in a state of light tension, producing "muscle tone". This keeps limbs and internal organs in their correct relative position. This should be an automatic result of imperceptible signals from receptors which indicate the condition and position of the muscles and organs.

When we have good posture, all voluntary muscles are lightly contracted, and none are over or under-contracted. But when we have bad posture, or slump, excess tension is placed on the lower back muscles, which will develop a nagging ache. At the same time, the organs in the abdomen are compressed as the spine and shoulders curve forward, reducing the efficiency of breathing and sometimes causing digestive upsets.

Cramp

Cramp is the most familiar muscular disorder, and results from a painful spasm or powerful sustained contraction of a muscle. It can be caused by a variety of factors. Salt deficiency can cause cramp, and this is common in hot climates, or among athletes. It is simply remedied by taking adequate salt in the diet, or by using salt tablets under exceptionally hot conditions, when much salt is lost through perspiration.

In people with poor circulation, due to the blood vessels leading to muscles "silting up", the reduced blood supply to the muscles often leads to painful cramp in the calves during walking. Even healthy people can suffer cramp after exertion (such as swimmer's cramp), probably due to the blood supply being reduced by spasms of the arteries in the limbs and back.

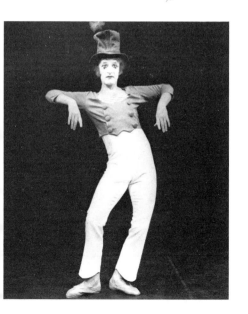

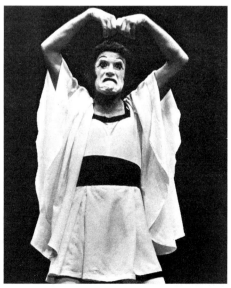

Blood

The 5½ litres (10 pints) or so of blood in the average adult body provide an essential link between all the tissues and organs of the body. Blood serves to transport food, oxygen and warmth where they are needed, and simultaneously, to remove waste products and carry them to the kidneys for elimination. As part of this continual work, the blood makes it possible for the body to identify invading organisms, destroy them, and remove their remains. It is a self-sealing liquid which, when it escapes through a wound, stops up the damaged area to prevent excessive losses.

All this takes place over an enormous distance, for when the total length of all the blood vessels of the body is added up, it reaches about 96,500 kilometres (60,000 miles).

All the blood in our bodies is pumped through the heart about 1,000 times each day, every day, until we die.

The components of blood

Blood is itself a tissue, with a number of separate components. Plasma is the liquid in which the other parts of the blood are carried. It consists of 92 per cent water, and smaller quantities of protein glucose, and other nutrients. It is the vehicle for the raw materials needed by the tissues. Plasma also carries hormones and various substances needed to fight infection and cause blood clotting.

The most plentiful components of the blood are red blood cells, which convey oxygen about the body. They are tiny discs, about 0.0762 mm (1/3,000 in) in diameter, and containing a substance called haemoglobin. Oxygen is picked up by red cells in the lungs, converting their contents to oxy-haemoglobin; the oxygen so incorporated is transported to the tissues of the body for release as required.

1 2 4 3 5

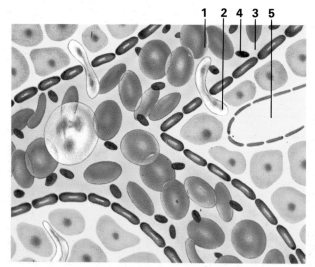

◀ Microscopic view of a blood capillary. The red cells (**1**) carry oxygen; the white cells (**2**) fight germs; the plasma (**3**) carries food, wastes and hormones and the platelets (**4**) help in clotting. From the capillary, oxygen and food pass to the surrounding cells. Part of the blood fluid also seeps out. This fluid, or lymph, bathes the nearby cells then drains back to the capillary or lymph channels (**5**).

▶ A cast of a baby's blood circulation

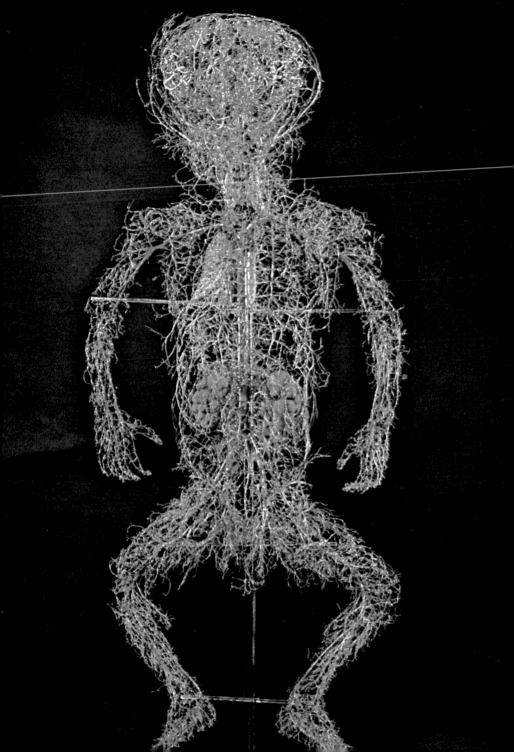

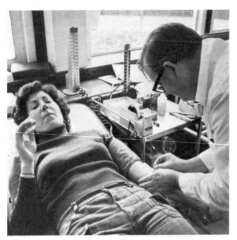

▲ Blood transfusion is a simple and painless procedure, which has saved countless lives. Donors can give blood several times each year without ill effects.

The blood also contains white blood cells, although these are fewer in number. Their functions are largely protective. Unlike red cells, they can squeeze through the walls of blood vessels into the surrounding tissues. White cells are of two basic types. Granulocytes respond rapidly to injury or infection, and congregate in the affected area. Lymphocytes, on the other hand, appear to be associated with immunity to infection, and respond quite slowly.

All of these blood cells, both red and white, are formed in bone marrow. Some white cells are also produced in the thymus gland, spleen, and lymph nodes, especially in response to an infection, when they may increase to 4 times their normal numbers.

Platelets

The other major constitutents of blood are platelets, or thrombocytes. These are tiny bodies produced by the bone marrow, and are present in huge numbers. They are responsible for clotting blood at the site of an injury. When a blood vessel is damaged, platelets in the immediate area stick to each other and to the wall of the vessel, until the aperture is sealed. Then fibrogen, a substance dissolved in plasma, produces thread-like stands of fibrin which enmesh the platelets, and eventually form a clot. With the gap temporarily sealed, the damaged tissues begin to regenerate.

Blood deficiencies

Because the blood is such an important transport system, reaching every part of the body, quite minor disturbances of its constituents can have serious effects.

Haemoglobin, the substance responsible for transporting oxygen to the other tissues, contains iron. If the diet is deficient in iron, the amount of haemoglobin in the red cells is diminished. The result is anaemia — a general weakness due largely to lack of oxygen in the tissues.

Allergies are another form of malfunction, resulting from inability of the body to distinguish harmless substances from potentially dangerous invaders. Antibodies are chemicals carried in the blood which inactivate foreign substances. But when antibodies are formed against harmless foods, clothing, or pollens, an allergy results. The body's response can be the cold-like symptoms of hay-fever, or itching and inflammation, or may sometimes be more serious, such as severe shock.

Immunisation

Antibodies are substances produced in the blood to combat bacteria and viruses. They develop naturally in the presence of infection, but the blood can be stimulated to produce antibodies by injecting dead or neutralised germs, or the toxins they produce, thus protecting against subsequent infection.

Transfusions

Our own red blood cells carry identifying substances which do not provoke a response from our own antibodies. But if blood from a person with a different blood group is transfused into our bloodstream, our system may react violently. Recognising transfused blood cells as invaders, our antibodies attack them, causing them to clump into groups which could rapidly block the blood vessels and cause death. This is why it is important to check the blood group before a transfusion.

Similarly, red cells may carry another substance called the Rhesus factor. A person *without* this factor is classed as having Rh-negative blood. If a woman has a child *with* the factor (Rh-positive) she may develop an antibody against the factor. Should a subsequent child be Rh-positive, her body can react so violently that the child must have its entire blood supply changed immediately after its birth, as it may otherwise die.

Leukaemia

Blood cells do not normally multiply. In leukaemia, however, which is a cancer-like disease, white cells have the ability to multiply, although they never reach full maturity. Consequently, the healthy white cells of the body are gradually replaced by the non-functioning leukaemic cells, leaving the patient with no defence against infection. The disease affects the bone marrow, and eventually the production of red cells is also affected, making the sufferer anaemic.

There are some promising new treatments which seem to provide a complete cure for some children suffering from leukaemia, although the adult form of the disease is more resistant to treatment.

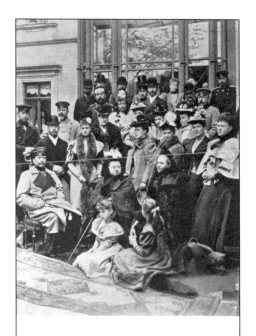

Queen Victoria, or possibly one of her ancestors, carried a mutated gene which devastated many of the Royal houses of Europe as her descendants interbred. This was the gene for haemophilia, which first became apparent in her sickly son, Leopold. He had serious haemorrhages from mild injuries, and died at age 31, but not before he had married and passed on the disease to his daughter. Girls are the unaffected carriers of haemophilia, and at least one of Victoria's daughters had already married and passed on the unsuspected condition. Most affected male children died young, so the disease tended to die out naturally. It is now probably extinct in the European royal families.

The vital organs

Contrary to popular belief, the heart is positioned almost exactly in the centre of the chest, although it is tilted slightly to the left. Throughout our lifetimes the heart beats tirelessly, about 75 times each minute. At times of stress it can speed up enormously, to as much as 250 beats per minute, but quickly returns to its normal rate. The sole purpose of the heart is to circulate blood around the body, against the resistance of the smallest blood vessels.

The heart is remarkably trouble-free for such a hard-working organ, but is subject to a number of congenital defects, and also to problems related to our hectic way of life.

The circulation system

Blood leaving the heart travels along arteries, which divide and divide again until they terminate in minute capillaries which infiltrate every organ in the body. These are so narrow that red blood cells have to squeeze through them. Oxygen in the red blood cells passes readily through the capillary walls into the tissues. At the same time, waste material, including carbon dioxide, passes out of the tissues into the blood. The deoxygenated blood in the capillaries now passes into a network of veins, which gradually come together into major vessels leading back to the heart. Veins differ from arteries in that they are thin-walled, with one-way valves to stop blood draining to the limbs when we stand erect. When these one-way valves are deficient, the veins in the legs become distended because of the excess pressure of blood. If they are near the skin, they produce varicose veins, which can be

In 1822, eighteen-year-old Alexis St Martin was accidentally shot in the chest by a musket, from a range of only three feet. The appalling wound was treated by pushing the lungs and stomach back, and hopefully closing the aperture with stitches. Against all expectation, he survived, and a week later was eating as normal. Except that most of what he ate came out through the remaining hole in his abdomen. In spite of this, he lived on, and the "window" in his stomach was the first insight into the workings of the digestive system. Through it, the actual process of digestion could be seen, and samples taken of digestive fluids.

removed surgically.

Because the capillaries and their associated blood vessels are so small, they produce resistance to the flow of blood, the source of blood pressure. This is what the doctor is measuring when he applies a sleeve to the arm and takes a reading from an attached gauge.

Hypertension

High blood pressure is one of the greatest killers of our time, as unless treated it can cause severe damage to the heart, kidneys, and brain. High blood pressure, or hyper-

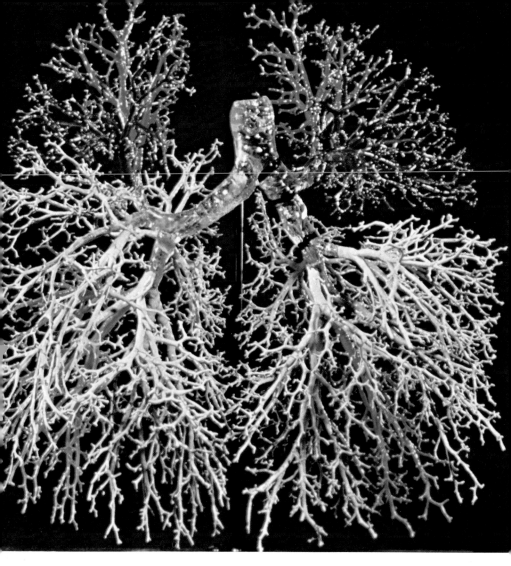

tension, seems to result from excessive constriction of the smallest blood vessels, the heart then having to work harder to force blood round the system. In response to these extra demands, it becomes enlarged, and may later fail completely. Similarly, the kidneys are unable to cope with the increased pressure, and as they fail, may make the hypertension worse.

With increasing age, the walls of arteries

▲ The lungs contain a delicate tracery of tiny blood vessels, here injected with a plastic material to show their structure.

lose their resilience, and if the blood pressure is sufficiently high, arteries supplying the brain may rupture, causing a stroke, with bleeding and damage which can be followed by paralysis or death.

The lungs

When we are resting, we breathe in about half a litre of air with each breath, and exhale the same quantity. But the air we breathe out has changed. It now contains less oxygen, and more carbon dioxide than the air we inhaled. The lungs fill the essential function of bringing air into near contact with blood, allowing the red blood cells to take in oxygen. At the same time carbon dioxide, a waste product, passes out of the blood and is exhaled.

Air enters the lungs through the nose and mouth, and passes down the trachea, an armoured flexible tube. This then subdivides into bronchi (the site of bronchitis) and smaller bronchioles, terminating in tiny bladders called alveoli. The alveoli are well supplied with blood vessels, and oxygen and carbon dioxide pass freely through their walls.

We inhale and exhale by two mechanisms. The rib cage can be expanded by muscles attached to the ribs and spine. This reduces the pressure in the lungs, causing air to enter. As the muscles relax, the rib cage contracts, forcing air out.

Additionally, breathing can be effected by the diaphragm; a sheet of muscle separating the lungs and heart from the organs in the abdomen. When it contracts, the volume of the rib cage increases, causing inhalation, followed by exhalation as it relaxes. Diaphragmic breathing is the most important form of respiration, breathing with the rib cage being used more during strenuous activity, when the body demands more oxygen.

Lung diseases

The delicate tissues lining the lungs are particularly prone to infection, and also to mechanical damage. The airways are lined with tiny beating hairs or cilia which cause a steady current of mucus to carry inhaled dust and other unwanted material out of the lungs and back to the throat, where it is periodically swallowed. Smoking paralyses these cilia, and allows mucus and the tar from cigarettes to accumulate in the lungs, causing "smoker's cough". Prolonged contact with these substances can give rise to lung cancer. Other substances can also evade the lung's defences, such as coal dust, asbestos fibres, and several other types of mineral dust, all capable of

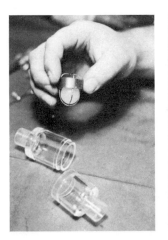
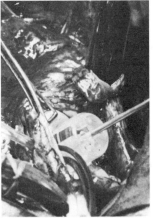

◀ When heart valves stop working through disease or damage, they can sometimes be replaced surgically. A heart-lung machine takes over the function of respiration, while the new valve is stitched into the open heart and the wound closed.

causing particular types of serious lung disease if inhaled over long periods.

The liver

The liver is the powerhouse for the entire body. It is the heaviest organ we possess, weighing about $1\frac{1}{2}$ kg, and is arranged in the upper abdomen, overlying the bulk of the intestines. The liver has several largely unrelated functions. It acts primarily as an energy store. One of the main products of digestion is glucose, which passes straight to the liver and is stored as glycogen until needed. When we undertake strenuous activity, glucose is needed by the muscles, so the liver converts glycogen back to glucose, under the influence of a hormone produced by the pancreas.

The liver contains the gall bladder, which empties bile into the duodenum through the bile duct. Bile is a greenish fluid which helps prepare fats for digestion, and is derived from red blood cells broken down by the liver.

Yet another of the liver's functions is to remove from the blood toxic substances, such as alcohol. It is this property of the liver which makes it vulnerable to damage in drug overdoses, or continual abuse in alcoholism, when it becomes fibrous or cirrhotic, or may even fail completely. It has remarkable powers of self-repair, but when severely damaged, jaundice results; the skin being yellow-coloured due to bile pigments in the blood.

The kidneys and bladder

All the cells in the body are living in an aquatic environment which we carry within us. Our cells are bathed in plasma from the blood, and even the cell contents are largely liquid. The function of the kidneys is to maintain this stable internal environment, removing waste materials, and en-

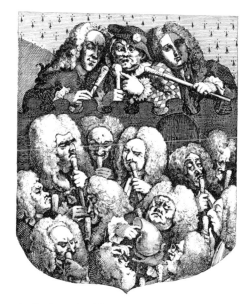

▲ During the 18th century, it was thought that most bodily ailments could be diagnosed by examining the urine of sick people. This satirical print shows doctors sniffing urine from a hollow cane.

suring that the proportions of the many chemicals in the blood remain constant.

The kidneys act as biological filters, capable of allowing only certain substances to pass. Blood entering the kidneys passes through a network of small blood vessels, where many of its constituents diffuse through the walls of the vessels into kidney tubules. Here, most of the water is re-absorbed, together with the nutrients, leaving concentrated liquid waste, or urine. In this way, they regulate the amount of water and other substances in the body.

Urine passes from the kidneys to the bladder, via a pair of tubes called ureters. In the bladder, urine is stored until increasing pressure warns us that the accumulated liquid must be voided, when it is passed out along the urethra.

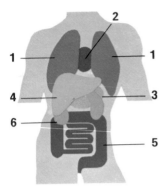

The vital organs

With the exception of the brain, all the vital organs of the body are housed in the trunk. This is divided into an upper and a lower region. In the upper trunk are the lungs; large paired spongy organs. The heart and the major blood vessels lie against the lungs, and all are surrounded and protected by the ribs, which also aid in breathing. In the lower abdomen are grouped the digestive system including the stomach, the liver, and the organs of excretion; the kidneys and bladder. Also in the lower abdomen are the sexual organs; testicles or ovaries.

1 Lungs
2 Heart
3 Stomach
4 Liver
5 Intestines
6 Kidneys

Dealing with alcohol

What happens when you drink a pint of beer, or a scotch? The alcohol it contains has an effect on the brain, but alcoholic drinks contain much else besides. The liquid passes rapidly down to the stomach (**1**) and the intestine (**2**). All the con-stituents of alcoholic drinks are soluble, so they can pass through the gut wall without being digested. The bloodstream carries all the constituents to the liver (**3**), where sugar is converted to glycogen and stored. Excess water passes in the bloodstream to the kidneys (**4**), then to the bladder (**5**) for excretion. The liver detoxifies most of the alcohol, and any remaining reaches the brain via the bloodstream (**6**).

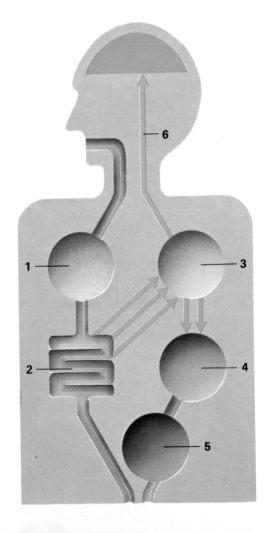

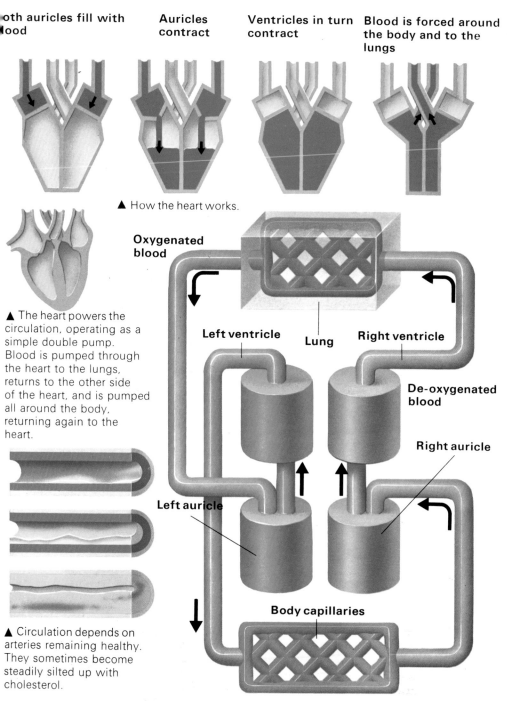

oth auricles fill with lood

Auricles contract

Ventricles in turn contract

Blood is forced around the body and to the lungs

▲ How the heart works.

Oxygenated blood

▲ The heart powers the circulation, operating as a simple double pump. Blood is pumped through the heart to the lungs, returns to the other side of the heart, and is pumped all around the body, returning again to the heart.

Left ventricle

Lung

Right ventricle

De-oxygenated blood

Right auricle

Left auricle

▲ Circulation depends on arteries remaining healthy. They sometimes become steadily silted up with cholesterol.

Body capillaries

The nervous system

The blood carrying its complex mixture of chemical messengers, or hormones, acts as a general communications network for the body. But for rapid control over movement, and to regulate the flow of hormones and other substances in the blood, a further system of communications is necessary.

The nervous system implements the orders of the brain, and keeps it constantly supplied with information as to the status of the body and its organs. Some of these activities do not require complex processing of information, and many are relegated to control by parts of the nervous system outside the brain. These are generally the routine activities and processes of the body, such as breathing, peristalstic movement in the intestines, and so on.

The autonomic nervous system

The spinal cord is an outgrowth of the brain, and contains grey and white matter in the same way as the brain. By operating a complex series of reflexes it is responsible for regulating many organs involved in respiration, the circulation of the blood, excretion, reproduction, and digestion. This part of the nervous system is called the autonomic nervous system, as it operates independently of conscious control. The central nervous system comprises the brain, and spinal nerves, and is ultimately responsible for the control of all activity.

The neuron

The whole complex network depends on the ability of a nerve cell to transmit a signal along its axon, or nerve fibre. Each neuron generates a minute electric charge, and when "switched-on" by a neighbouring neuron, the charge travels rapidly along the fibre, like a fuse burning towards a detonator. When the signal reaches the branched end of the fibre, it causes the release of a chemical that crosses the small gap separating one nerve cell from another. This chemical triggers the next fibre—or fibres—in the circuit. Each neuron is capable of producing only one response—a simple on or off signal, so the difference in the pain we experience when pricked with a pin or struck violently results only from variation in the number of neurons being stimulated or the frequency with which they are firing.

The tiny nerve fibres are extremely fragile, and are easily put out of action.

Nerves are a biological equivalent of electrical wiring and pass very small electrical signals along their conducting core, by a complex chemical process. The "insulation" of the nerve fibre is the myelin sheath which surrounds the axon for most of its length. When this covering breaks down, signals can no longer be passed effectively. In multiple sclerosis, the myelin sheath is destroyed, and signals can no longer be passed to muscles, which become progressively weaker. Very recently, it has been found that a virus may cause this breakdown, and it is likely that a vaccine could be developed to help fight the disease.

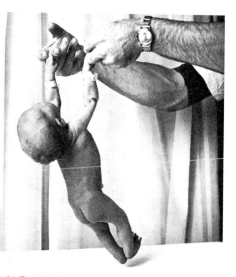

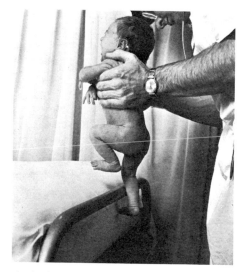

▲ For the first two months of life, babies have a "grasp reflex". When their palm is touched, the hand grips convulsively, so strongly that the baby can support its own weight while clinging to a finger.

▲ A similar reflex causes a new-born baby to make a walking movement when held with its feet resting lightly on the ground and moved forward, although it cannot support any weight. This reflex disappears after 6 weeks.

The numbness we experience after sitting awkwardly for too long is the result of pressure on a nerve, which is a bundle of nerve fibres. When the pressure is relieved, we feel tingling as the recovering nerve fibres fire off random signals.

Diseases of the nervous system

Many of the larger nerve fibres have a covering layer of insulating material called the myelin sheath. In many diseases of the nervous system it is damage to this myelin sheath which causes the efficiency of the nervous system to drop, as signals can no longer be transmitted so effectively. Diseases such as multiple sclerosis, diptheria, and alcoholism all damage the myelin sheath. Lesser diseases such as neuralgia are caused by inflammation of a nerve, while in shingles, a virus attacks the nerve, causing severe and prolonged discomfort.

Severe damage to the spine puts pressure on the spinal cord, or may even sever it. The results are paralysis of those parts of the body below the damage. Usually, however, the reflexes of the autonomic nervous system are still intact, so the vital processes of the body are still carried out, although the injured person has no sensation or voluntary control over most of his body.

The reflex arc

The simplest form of reflex involves only three neurons of the 12 thousand million neurons in the body. They work in a simple sequence. When a receptor anywhere in the body receives a stimulus, a signal is transmitted along the axon to a sensory neuron, which is usually situated in a ganglion, or small swelling in a nerve.

From here, the signal is passed on to an association neuron in the spinal cord, which sends out a further signal to a motor or secretory neuron. This neuron then conveys a signal to the appropriate part of the body, producing a response.

In practice, this means that when we touch a hot surface, or prick ourselves with a pin, the consequent reflex arc makes us move our hand away without reference to the brain. As all the information is processed by the spinal cord, an appropriate response can be made immediately. A split second later, a message from pain receptors on the skin reaches the brain, but by then, the muscles have already acted. Normally many more than three neurons are involved in this activity, as quite complex movements must be made to avoid a painful stimulus.

A similar reflex arc takes place when the tendon below the knee-cap is tapped. This contains receptors which measure the amount of tension on the muscle. When the tendon is tapped sharply, the receptors feed false information to the spinal cord and back to the muscle, causing the leg to jerk.

The reflex arc

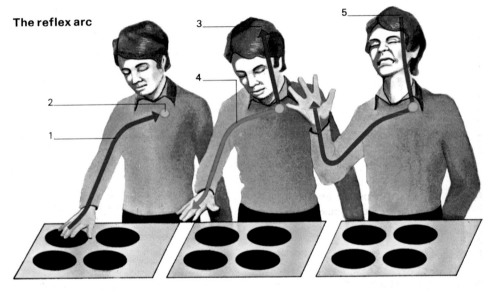

▲ When we touch a hot object, our body moves into action faster than the brain can react. Tiny receptors in the skin register the sensation of heat (or of any other potentially damaging stimulus), and rapidly pass a signal via nerves (**1**) to a swelling in the spinal cord, called a ganglion (**2**).

▲ From the ganglion, two signals are produced. One passes up the spinal cord to the brain (**3**), informing it of the potentially dangerous situation. The other message is fed back to muscles (**4**) powering the limb, causing them to contract violently and whisk the finger away.

▲ By the time we realise that the finger has been burned, and the brain registers pain (**5**), the hand is out of harm's way. This is an involuntary action, and the process controlling it is called a reflex arc. It is an important protective mechanism for the body. The "blink reflex" protects the delicate surface of the eye.

The brain

The most complex mechanism known to exist is a double-handful of tissue with the consistency of cold porridge. Our brains are capable of calculations more rapid than those of the fastest computer, yet can carry them out without our exerting any conscious effort.

When we step into a busy road and dodge traffic as we cross, our brains are computing continuously; noting our own speed and position, and the speed and position of a large number of other pedestrians and vehicles, then issuing detailed instructions to the body to allow us to cross without accident. Compare this to the "brain" of a guided missile, which usually only has to deal with a single moving target. Yet our brains can simultaneously cope with hundreds of variable "targets".

But the brain is much more than a complex computer. It has a unique ability to think, and to produce emotion. The brain is the seat of consciousness, and is where "we" reside—the home of the soul. Any or all of the organs of the body could be removed, but if the brain were kept alive, "we" would still be conscious of our existence. This terrifying experiment has actually been carried out on the isolated brains of dogs and monkeys, which have survived for long periods when separated from their bodies.

Brain waves

It is possible to measure the activity of the brain by means of tiny electrical currents which continually flicker across its surface. These can be detected even through the bones of the skull and the skin, by means of wires attached to an electro-encephalograph (EEG) machine. In the experiment just mentioned, the EEG showed that the isolated brains, connected to the blood supply of another animal, were actually "thinking".

Electrical energy is the key to the brain and how it works. The brain does not appear very complex when examined by the eye. It has various well-defined areas, and two obvious layers; an outer layer of *grey matter,* and an inner layer of *white matter*. These layers contain neurons, all essentially the same in structure. They have a rounded "body" (the grey matter of the brain), out of which a long thread or axon emerges (lying in the white matter).

Phineas Gage was a railroad builder in the U.S.A., when in 1848 he was tamping down a gunpowder charge in a hole drilled in the rock obstructing the route. He tamped too hard; the charge exploded, and blew the metre long steel bar, over 20 mm thick, up through his jaw, and out of the top of his head. Although a large amount of his brains had been blown out, Gage didn't lose consciousness, and walked unassisted to the doctor. He recovered without event, except for blindness in one eye, caused by a severed nerve. His character had changed drastically, however, and this gave neurosurgeons the clue to the physical basis for personality.

Signals or impulses are carried along these axons, until they reach the branched endings which contact other neurons.

Here they pass the signal on, and cause these neurons in turn to produce signals, rather like ripples spreading from a stone thrown into a pond. These electrical ripples spread out across the brain's surface, producing the wave-like patterns or rhythms which are detected by the EEG machine. They are the actual patterns of thought, or rather, of mental activity. When we are deep in thought, jagged spikes of electrical activity are recorded on the EEG machine, while when resting or asleep, we revert to a regular wave-like pattern.

The brain map

The electrical activity of the brain provides the key to the functioning of its different areas. By inserting tiny electrodes into the brain at different points, and applying very small electrical currents, a patient can experience apparently normal functioning of that segment of brain. If the current is applied to a motor area, it may cause a finger to twitch, or a limb to jerk. In the area concerned with hearing, the subject may mentally "hear" an actual sound. Some of the oddest effects have been the revealing of almost forgotten events, which unroll like a film when a particular spot on the brain is stimulated, and vanish when the current is switched off.

While many areas of the brain can be mapped by these means, other larger parts have no apparent function. Indeed, large sections of brain can be destroyed by accident or surgery with very little apparent effect. So division of work within the brain is an extremely flexible affair. Memories seem to be permanently imprinted on certain parts of the brain like the magnetic trace in a tape recording, but so prodigious is the brain's capacity to store information that only a fraction of the available storage area can be filled in a lifetime. Our intellectual capacity far exceeds our ability to live on to exploit it.

Sleep—the unconscious mind

We spend about a third of our lives asleep, but this period is only a time of physical rest. While we sleep, our brains are extremely active, as can be shown by EEG records of the sleeping brain.

Sleeping brain activity is closely associ-

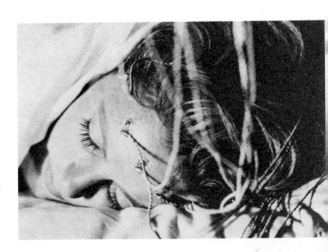

► Electroencephalogram or EEG being taken. This monitors the general pattern of electrical activity of many millions of nerve cells discharging minute electrical impulses. It has been suggested that it is possible for people to "tune into" the pleasurable alpha waves by practicing with this machine and thereby consciously control their mental state.

Awake and relaxed

Awake and concentrating

Ordinary sleep

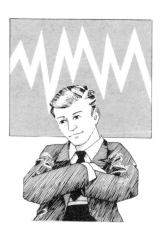

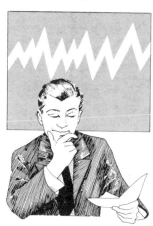

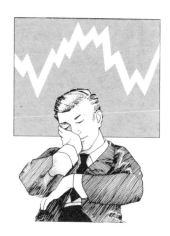

▲ A regular pattern of wave-like electrical discharges plays over the brain.

▲ While concentrating hard, jagged discharges show our brain is at work.

▲ During sleep, a different, pattern of waves is produced depending on the depth of sleep.

ated with dreaming. Although we are not usually aware of it, we all dream four or five times each night, for a total of nearly an hour. During dreaming, the brain produces unusual electrical signals, and distinct physical changes take place in the rest of the body. Our muscles become totally relaxed, while our eyes move about rapidly beneath the closed eyelids.

This period of rapid eye movement, or REM sleep, is very important to our well-being. If people are deprived of REM sleep by being constantly awakened each time they begin to dream, they begin to show various mental abnormalities, and may suffer hallucinations. When they are finally allowed to sleep undisturbed they dream almost continuously for a while, making up their missed "dreamtime". Babies have REM sleep most of the time, and it diminishes as we grow older.

Freud and his successors believe that dreaming exposes our innermost feelings, but other psychologists think that this is simply the brain's way of disposing of unwanted or out-dated information; rather like re-programming a computer.

Brain transmitters

Although electrical energy powers the brain, this is generated by chemical means. Electrical signals are passed from one nerve fibre to the next by means of chemical messenger substances or neuro-transmitters. The quantities of these substances present in the body are so small as to be almost unmeasurable, but they affect our behaviour in many fundamental ways.

It has been found that neuro-transmitter substance is deficient in the brains of people suffering from depression, and modern anti-depressant drugs help to restore the normal chemical balance. If there is too much transmitter substance, a person may be in a continual state of excitement, and this situation has been found in several serious mental disorders.

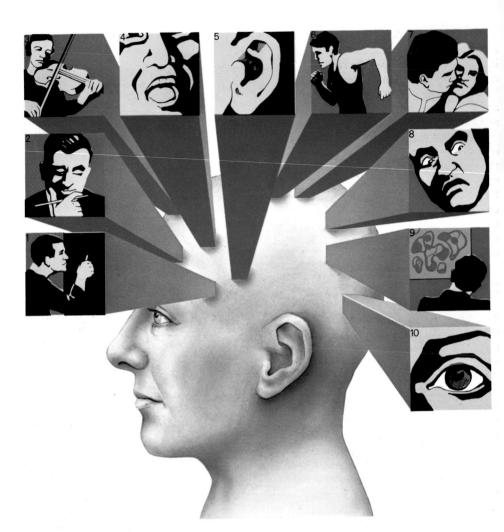

The areas of the brain
1 Perceptual judgement
2 Thinking
3 Movement and planning
4 Speech
5 Hearing
6 Movement
7 Sensation
8 Sensory analysis
9 Visual interpretation
10 Sight

The brain is often likened to a computer, but is vastly more complex. Although it uses electrical signals to communicate with the rest of the body, its "wiring" is so complicated that there is a wide choice of path for each signal. There are few obvious structures in the brain, but different functions are controlled by particular areas. Between these areas, pathways of nerves provide connections and allow us to correlate the signals we receive from the world around us. We see, hear, taste, smell, and touch our environment continuously, and different parts of the brain assess each of these inputs independently.

Even the humble cup of coffee or tea affects the transmitter substances. Caffeine in these drinks increases the rate of release of the transmitter, and gives us a mental "lift". More powerful stimulants like amphetamines have a similar but much more powerful effect.

A whole range of drugs have dramatic effects on the brain. The best-known and the most powerful of these is LSD which causes hallucinations. It is not known how these drugs work on the brain, but chemically, most are very similar to the transmitter substances, and probably trick the brain into using them, rather than the correct transmitter.

Disorders of the brain

The brain is in other ways a delicate structure. It needs large quantities of nutrients and oxygen to maintain its efficiency, and can survive for only a few minutes if the blood supply is cut off. It ceases to work effectively within seconds if the supply is temporarily checked, as by pressure on the arteries of the neck. Unlike almost all the other tissues of the body, nervous tissue cannot regenerate after injury, so when brain cells start to die off due to failing blood supplies in old age, the loss is permanent, often resulting in mental confusion and senility.

Other mental disturbances have no obvious cause, although this is a matter of dispute among some researchers, who feel that mental illness may be due to chemical changes in the body. A few mental disturbances result from known diseases, such as syphilis, meningitis, encephalitis, or brain tumours, but most seem to arise spontaneously, perhaps caused by external factors.

Epilepsy is a fairly common disorder resulting when electrical activity on the brain's surface is uncontrolled, sending an electrical storm of discharges across the brain, and causing convulsions. Lesser disorders such as headaches are occasionally caused by irritation of the membranes covering the brain, although the brain itself is almost totally insensitive, and brain surgery can be carried out on a conscious patient with only a local anaesthetic.

Migraine is a mysterious disorder which may be connected with the functioning of the brain. Its causes are uncertain, but may be due to spasms of the small arteries in the brain and around the head.

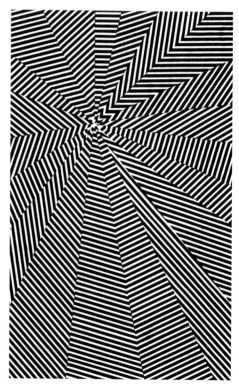

▲ Migraine attacks are often preceded by interference with vision. This is an impression of the pattern often seen by sufferers just before a migraine attack.

Sensing the world

Our appreciation of the outside world is assessed by the brain, which at the same time receives information from sense organs monitoring conditions inside the body. Receptors in the muscles and tendons measure the position of the body and limbs, and organs in the ear note the movements of the head. Other receptors monitor the activity of internal organs.

Touch

Within the skin are specialised nerve endings, each of which registers either touch, pressure, pain, heat, or cold. The degree to which we experience the sensation depends on how many of these receptors are stimulated. A person insensitive to pressure or pain is lucky to survive childhood, for when they grip anything they are liable to break their fingers by squeezing too hard. Sprains, broken bones, and worst of all, severe burns, take a heavy toll of those with a deficient sense of touch.

Taste and smell

Taste and smell are not very important to humans, although they have a very real function in stimulating the digestive system when we begin to eat. Our sense of taste is poorly developed; we only recognise four different tastes—sweet, sour, salt and bitter. Taste is a so-called "chemical sense", which depends on the

▼ Our senses are much more efficient than we realise. When one sense is damaged or lost, other senses sharpen to compensate. With practice, blind people can learn to read Braille with their finger-tips.

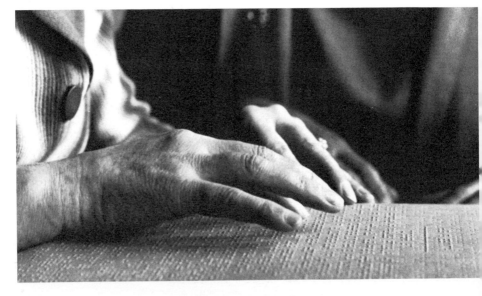

substance placed in the mouth dissolving slightly in the saliva. Anything which does not dissolve will not have any taste.

Most of the flavour we experience when eating is smell, rather than taste, for tiny particles of food rise in the back of the mouth and pass into the nasal passage. Here these food particles, or substances inhaled through the nose, dissolve in the film of mucus within the nasal cavity, and stimulate olfactory receptors. These are much more sensitive than the receptors on the tongue, and are capable of identifying minute amounts of substances in the air we breathe—even when they are diluted to 1 part in 50,000 million.

Hearing

Unlike taste and smell, hearing is based on mechanical stimulation of receptors. The exact mechanism is not fully understood, for the ear can detect a much wider range of sounds than would be expected. The loudest sound we can record is a million times louder than the quietest. Our brain selects the sounds it wishes to "hear", and rejects the rest, so we can follow one person's conversation in a roomful of chattering people.

Sight

The eyes are our single most important sense. They are situated well to the front of the skull, to give us binocular vision, and are sunk in slightly so that the ridge of bone behind the eyebrows protects them from accident.

Because the eyes are so complex, minor malfunctions cause serious problems. With increasing age, the resilient lens becomes harder, and the muscles of the eye are unable to distort it sufficiently to focus. When this happens, bifocal lensed spectacles are usually prescribed. These allow one section of the glass to be used for close work, while the rest of the lens is ground so as to allow normal vision of more distant objects. Other disabilities like long or short-sightedness result from developmental faults in the eye.

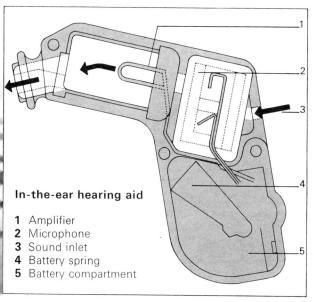

In-the-ear hearing aid

1 Amplifier
2 Microphone
3 Sound inlet
4 Battery spring
5 Battery compartment

◀ When deafness results from a thickened ear drum, or from a disorder of the tiny bones conducting sound within the ear, a hearing aid can often help restore almost full use of the ears. This simple electronic device picks up sound waves via a tiny microphone, amplifies them, and plays them back into the canal leading into the ear mechanism.

The sense organs

We maintain our awareness of the outside world by means of sense organs. Without senses, our brains would be useless. We would have no knowledge, and would be unable to learn. Sense organs are grouped about the body in strategic areas. The organs of touch reflect the importance of the areas in which they are grouped. If a plan is drawn of the body, with the sizes of the various parts drawn in proportion to the importance of the sense organs, it produces the "homunculus" shown below. This shows how sensitive are the lips, feet, and particularly, the hands.

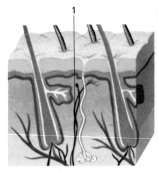

One function of the skin is to act as a large and complex sense organ. Throughout the skin run many nerves (**1**) and nerve endings which are capable detecting a wide range of stimuli. Touch, pressure, pain, warmth, and cold can all be perceived as separate sensations, and more specialised sensations such as wetness or stickiness result from a combination of these.

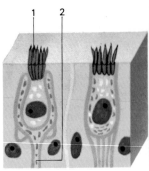

The ear transmits sound vibrations from the ear drum, via tiny bones to the cochlea, where sensory hairs (**1**) register vibration and send messages along nerves (**2**) to the brain.

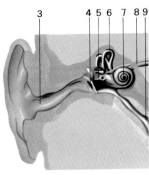

3 Ear canal, **4** Ear drum, **5** 3-bone lever, **6** Semi-circular canals (balance), **7** Cochlea, **8** Auditory nerve, **9** Eustachian tube.

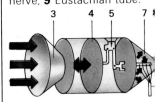

The ear is an amplifier, turning sound vibrations into electrical signals.

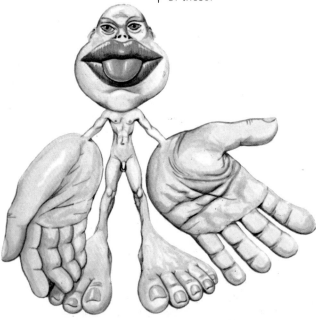

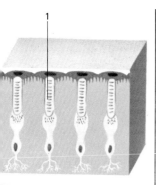

The retina is the screen at the back of the eyeball, on which light is focussed by the lens. Images are picked up by rods (**1**) and cones; special cells which can detect changes in light intensity.

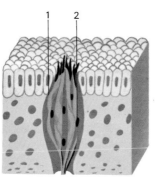

Taste is one of the chemical senses, detecting small amounts of substances dissolved in the saliva. Taste buds (**1**) on the tongue contain gustatory cells (**2**) which detect sweet, sour, salt and bitter tastes.

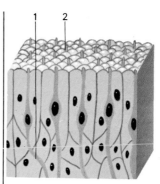

Much of what we perceive as 'taste' is actually smell, caused when tiny food particles rise into the nasal region. Nerves (**1**) receive signals from receptor cells (**2**) which are stimulated by substances dissolved in a mucus layer.

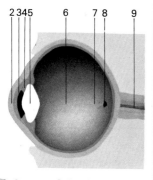

2 Cornea, **3** Pupil, **4** Iris, **5** Lens, **6** Vitreous humour, **7** Retina, **8** Blind spot, **9** Optic nerve.

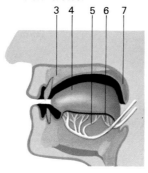

3 Hard palate, **4** Papillae, **5** Lingual nerve, **6** Glossopharyngeal nerve, **7** Soft palate.

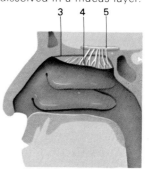

3 Ethmoid palate, **4** Olfactory membrane, **5** Olfactory bulb.

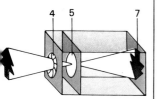

The eye operates much like a camera, producing an inverted image on the retina.

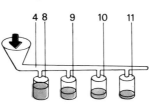

Flavour is built up from the four simple tastes; sweet (**8**), sour (**9**), bitter (**10**), and salt (**11**).

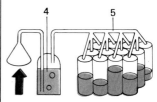

The sense of smell resembles that of taste, but is immensely more sensitive.

Skin

Our skin provides protection for the delicate tissues of the body. It gives some mechanical protection against cuts and blows, and at the same time prevents the loss of too much water by evaporation.

But the skin does much more than this. It is a complex organ in its own right. While it prevents excess water loss, it does allow the escape of some water for particular functions. When the body overheats as a result of violent activity or excessively hot weather, the skin secretes perspiration through its 2½ million sweat glands. As this evaporates on the surface

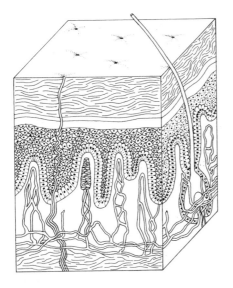

▲ The skin is the largest of the body's organs, and is an extremely complex device to protect our surface, control body temperature, and to remove some waste material in the form of perspiration. All the skin cells visible on the surface are dead, and being replaced by live cells beneath.

of the skin, it cools the body.

Sun and skin

Because our conventions of beauty decree that some degree of skin colouring is desirable, many of us spend a great deal of money and time in ensuring that we are exposed to as much sun as possible. This increases the amount of melanin pigment present in the skin which is produced by the body as a defence against excess ultraviolet radiation in the sun's light. Without this protection, the skin will become severely burned and blistered. Melanin develops only slowly, so gradual exposure to sunlight allows a protective tan to build up without risk of sunburn. Albinos lack this pigment, so their skin remains pink and delicate at all times. Apart from its cosmetic effect, sunlight also produces most of the vitamin D needed by the body.

Skin layers

The hair which covers most of our body, some coarse, some fine, is a residue from our evolutionary past. It now has little protective function, and the oil or sebum which is secreted by sebaceous glands was once used to make hair partly water-repellant. Now, however, it serves to keep skin pliable, and together with the perspiration, acts as a mild antiseptic. Neither sebum nor perspiration has any noticeable smell, and "B.O." occurs solely as a result of bacteria acting on the secretions. Simple washing, if done frequently, is enough to prevent this odour.

Skin is built up in several layers, and the outer layer consists of dead cells which are continually being sloughed off and replaced. The inner layer, or dermis, contains tough connective tissue, which gives the skin its elastic strength, and is richly supplied with blood vessels and touch receptors.

Hair

Hair, like the nails, is an outgrowth of the skin, with a protective function. Hairs grow from small pits or follicles in the skin, lubricated by sebaceous glands. The hair is itself dead tissue, and the hairdresser's description of "lifeless hair" is appropriate to even the healthiest scalp. With increasing age, the tubular hairs often contain air pockets and this causes grey hair. Dry hair results from an inadequate supply of sebum from the sebaceous glands, and conversely, oily hair is caused by their overactivity.

Shaving and hair removal is popularly supposed to cause the hair to grow more vigorously, but in fact has no effect whatsoever—it simply makes the stubble remaining feel more bristly. The amount of body hair we have is controlled by hormones, and in women near their menopause, changes in the balance of hormones in the blood can cause unwanted facial hair to appear. Treatment with female hormones usually reverses this process, however.

The causes of balding and falling hair are not known, though they may relate to poor blood supply to the hair follicles. In practice, we are continually losing hair and replacing it with fresh growth. The 120,000 hairs on the scalp grow about $\frac{1}{3}$ mm each day.

Nails

Nails are simply fused hairs, and are composed of the same material, keratin. They have little real function in humans, except to protect the finger tips, but

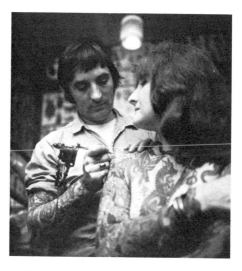

▲ Decoration of the skin by tatooing is an ancient art, carried out by injecting insoluble pigment under the skin. Removing the colour can be a long and painful process.

remain as a legacy from our past.

They are particularly liable to show growth defects, which appear as a ridge or white fleck. Many illnesses cause this kind of mark, and malnutrition can also contribute. Iron deficiency makes the growing nails thin and soft, and this frequently occurs during pregnancy.

Skin disorders

All parts of the skin are growing rapidly. Epidermal cells, hair, nails, and sweat glands are liable to diseases and disorders characteristic of fast-growing tissue. Eczema is an inflamatory disease, in which too many epidermal cells are produced, causing blisters and scales on the surface.

Various other conditions, such as blackheads, are caused by the blocking of sweat glands and follicles, and when the trapped material becomes infected, boils or acne can follow.

The digestion system

Our digestive systems operate like complex chemical works which allow our bodies to make use of the food we eat. Food cannot enter our systems unless it is broken down into simple molecules which are small enough to pass through the walls of the intestine and enter the bloodstream. In the process of digestion this breakdown takes place in a number of simple stages, each controlled by enzymes: chemicals produced by the body which act as catalysts. These speed up the process.

Throughout its entire length of thirty or more feet, the digestive system conveys food through a tube lined with delicate tissues, which could be readily digested by the corrosive liquids they contain. Our tissues are almost identical to those of the animals we eat, yet our bodies digest animal proteins while simultaneously protecting us from the same process. When this protection breaks down, the result is digestive disorder.

Upsets in the system

Any process as complicated as digestion is liable to malfunction. Even some of the body's normal functions can affect digestion. Under stress conditions for instance the peristaltic action of the intestine to falter. The muscle tone of the entire digestive system is reduced, and the stomach literally sags. The walls of the intestine lose their normal healthy pink colour, and become pale and flabby. If the stress conditions continue, digestive upsets result. Poor digestion, nausea, and diarrhoea can all be caused by emotional stress. Equally, if peristalsis is too rapid,

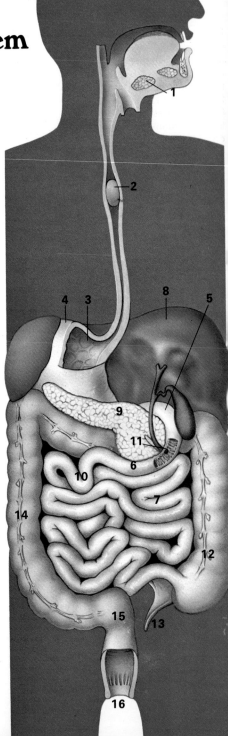

Digestion starts in the mouth, where food is cut and ground by the chewing action of the teeth, and moistened with saliva from the saliva gland (**1**) to make it easy to swallow. Saliva contains an enzyme called ptyalin, which breaks down starches into sugars which can be readily absorbed.

Pyloric sphincter

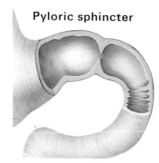

the food are finally broken down into a size which can be absorbed. This is aided by the presence of villi (**11**) over the intestinal lining. These are tiny finger-like projections which increase the area of the intestinal surface, allowing more of the digested material to be absorbed.

Stomach wall

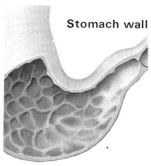

From the mouth, food (**2**) is pushed down the oesophagus by a wave-like muscular movement called peristalsis, which propels food right through the digestive system. When it reaches the stomach (**3**), digestion begins in earnest. The stomach is a large muscular organ in which food is churned up with a variety of digestive fluids. It secretes hydrochloric acid, which works with an enzyme called pepsin to break down protein into simpler substances. To prevent this potent liquid attacking the stomach wall (**4**), large quantities of protective mucus are produced. When this stage of digestion is complete, the food is discharged through a muscular valve,

the sphincter (**5**), into the duodenum (**6**), which is the first part of the small intestine.

As the food passes along the intestine (**7**), it is flooded with a succession of enzymes and other substances which aid their action. Bile for example, is a liquid produced by the liver (**8**), which breaks down fats into tiny globules. These globules are more easily attacked by enzymes such as those produced in the pancreas (**9**). This is a large gland which not only produces enzymes, but also liberates the hormone insulin directly into the blood stream.

In the small intestine (**10**) the complex molecules in

Pancreas

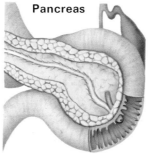

Once absorbed, the nutrients enter the tiny capillary vessels and are carried through the body in the bloodstream. However, not all the food is digested, and the remains must be removed. As this material leaves the small intestine, it passes through the caecum (**12**), to which the appendix (**13**) is attached. The liquid waste is passed into the colon (**14**),

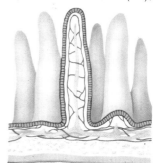

Villi of small intestine

where any remaining nutrients are absorbed, and water is removed to solidify the remaining material. This passes through the last part of the system, the rectum (**15**), and leaves the body through the anus (**16**), as faeces.

faeces will be passed before the excess fluid can be removed, and again, this will cause diarrhoea.

Some digestive disorders are widely misunderstood. Heartburn, for example, usually results when air is swallowed while eating too rapidly. This bubbles back up the oesophagus, carrying with it some of the stomach acid, and causing a burning sensation in the chest. Similarly, stomach acid is a natural condition rather than a disorder, although the manufacturers of antacids have convinced us that it should be "treated".

Some problems are caused by the actual structure of the digestive system. The appendix, for example, is a finger-like bag leading off the gut, and it is inevitable that this will sometimes trap partly-digested food. With the profusion of bacteria inhabiting the gut, this trapped material is liable to become putrid, causing appendicitis. Any bacterial infection of the intestine wall results in abdominal discomfort, as the intestinal fluids attack the damaged tissues and the whole complex sequence of digestion is upset.

A spoonful of roughage

Some problems are caused directly by faulty diets. Constipation, for example, is a dietary problem of "civilised" man. Our digestive system is adapted by evolution to deal with a diet consisting mostly of vegetable material, which can be only incompletely digested. The bulky waste remaining stimulates the colon to pass faeces quite frequently. But modern man eats a diet of refined food which can be almost entirely digested. The small bulk of waste is insufficient to stimulate the colon to remove the material and causes constipation. This is simply rectified by eating foods containing roughage such as bran, but if the condition is allowed to continue,

even more uncomfortable disorders may occur, such as haemorrhoids.

Some medical researchers believe that diseases like bowel cancer are triggered off by our low-bulk diets. When faeces remain in the gut for a long period, the bacteria living in the gut feed on this waste material and may produce toxins which could cause cancer.

Processed indigestion

Modern "scientific" diets are suspected of causing a great deal of the intestinal illnesses now so common. Our digestive systems are remarkably efficient in coping with diets ranging from blood and milk in the Masai tribes of Africa, to fish and

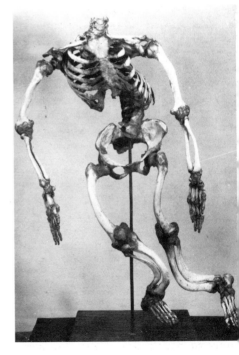

▲ Rickets causes severe skeletal deformities. Curved bones and swollen joints may remain even after the vitamin deficiency is corrected.

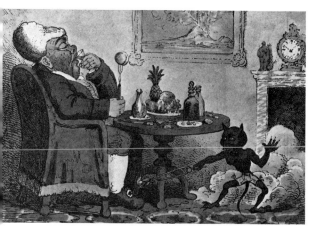

◀ Gout is often thought to be amusing, but is one of the most painful diseases known. It is a disorder of the metabolism, and the pain is caused by the accumulation of tiny crystals of uric acid in the joints. This may be influenced by the diet. Kidney, liver, and vegetables like peas all contain chemicals which could cause gout.

whale blubber among eskimos, and almost pure rice diets in many people living in the Far East. Yet these are all "natural" diets, for which we were evolutionarily designed. But if you look at the list of ingredients on any pack of processed food, you will find a large number of materials which we are not designed to cope with. In particular, chemical food additives have given rise to concern. Processed food contains colourants, preservatives, flavourings, chemicals to improve the consistency of the food, and a whole range of other sophisticated products of the food technologist's art. All are supposedly safe, but this is difficult to prove.

The normal gut is protected from its corrosive contents by a thick layer of mucus. If this is breached by infections or stress interfering with intestinal function, the results can be serious. As the digestive enzymes attack the intestinal wall, small ulcers are produced. These start as pits in the intestinal lining, but as the acid and enzymes eat deeper, they reach the unprotected muscle layers. First the ulcer bleeds into the gut, then, may perforate, releasing the gut contents into the body cavity and causing severe shock and even death. But if an ulcer is recognised early,

and a sensible diet is followed, it will usually clear up rapidly.

Diet deficiencies

Bad diets can have both temporary and long-term effects on our health. We all recognise indigestion as the immediate result of faulty eating habits, but prolonged dietary deficiencies have more insidious effects. We are familiar with the results of prolonged famine in the overpopulated areas of the world, but the diseases we now see on news broadcasts were once common in our own countries.

Protein deficiency can lead to kwashiorkor, a disease which produces the pot-bellied, spindly-limbed children recently seen in Biafra and Bangladesh. Rickets is another deficiency disease which still occurs among the socially underpriviledged in even the most developed countries. It is caused by a deficiency of Vitamin D. This vitamin D is produced in the skin by sunlight, or can be obtained from fresh food. Rickets was particularly common among children working in poorly-lit factories during the Industrial Revolution, subsisting on an inadequate diet, and seldom seeing the sun.

Glands

In a sense, man is the prisoner of his glands. Our emotions, reactions, and behaviour are as much controlled by glands as by the nervous system. The body contains a complex, interlinked network of glands, which work closely with the nervous system in maintaining the human machine.

Our skin is covered with sweat glands: tiny tube-like structures which are clustered in areas like the under-arm region, the pubic area, face, hands and feet. They serve the dual purpose of removing waste from the blood and keeping the body cool, for as the sweat evaporates from the skin, it produces a drop in temperature. Use of deodorants which constrict the sweat glands can make you feel warmer, though less "sticky".

Other glands help with the digestion, and the most apparent of these are the salivary glands in the mouth. They provide a good example of how the function of glands is associated with the nervous system. The sight of food is often sufficient for the brain to activate the salivary glands, as the first step in digestion. Other glands of similar type line the digestive system, all producing chemicals to help break down food.

All of these glands, whether opening on the body surface or pouring out their secretions through a duct, are known as exocrine glands. The other major group are the endocrine glands, which empty directly into the bloodstream.

Chemical messengers

The endocrine glands produce hormones, or chemical messengers, which "switch on" or "turn off" other organs in the same way as does the nervous system. They are present in the blood in very small but

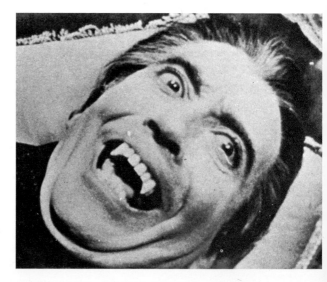

► When we watch a horror film, our body goes through all the changes associated with fear. Our hair prickles; we feel first hot, then cold; our heart races, and our mouth feels dry. But the brain is not truly frightened. Because we know that we are in no personal danger, we can allow ourselves the luxury of enjoying the sensation of fear and panic. Adrenalin, like many other drugs, acts as a strong stimulant, though produced by the body itself.

precisely measured quantities, and the balance of hormones in the bloodstream determines our mental and physical state.

When we are frightened or angry, we are in the grip of a complex glandular and nervous reaction. We see something which stimulates the brain to react with a "fight or flight" reaction. This activates the pituitary gland, a tiny pea-like organ situated deep within the brain, and the pituitary immediately frees a hormone into the blood. This is rapidly carried in the bloodstream to the adrenal glands, small bean-shaped organs near the kidneys.

The pituitary hormone "switches on"

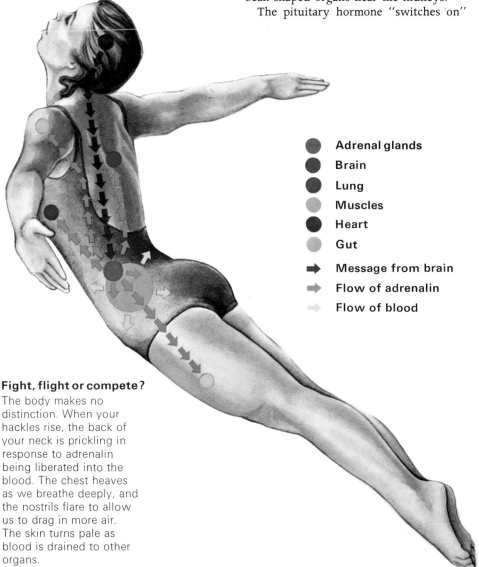

● Adrenal glands
● Brain
● Lung
● Muscles
● Heart
● Gut
➡ Message from brain
➡ Flow of adrenalin
➡ Flow of blood

Fight, flight or compete?
The body makes no distinction. When your hackles rise, the back of your neck is prickling in response to adrenalin being liberated into the blood. The chest heaves as we breathe deeply, and the nostrils flare to allow us to drag in more air. The skin turns pale as blood is drained to other organs.

the adrenals, so that they in turn produce adrenalin, a very powerful hormone. As this passes into the bloodstream, it causes all the body changes we associate with fear and anger. The heart is stimulated, and pumps more rapidly, and at the same time, our lungs work more efficiently. When we are readied for sudden exertion, the muscles will need the maximum amount of oxygen, so the blood supply to the intestine is temporarily checked, to make more blood available elsewhere. Exertion will burn up energy, so glucose is released into the blood.

The body is now keyed up and ready for action, either from fear and anger, or as a result of excitement. To some extent, this is an involuntary action, but for the athlete, it is essential that these hidden reserves are utilised. The period of winding up before an athletic event is intended to give the body time to reach this peak condition.

Glandular disorders

The glands controlling our bodies can malfunction in a number of ways. The secretions from the adrenal glands are intended to ready us to escape from unpleasant situations, or to fight. But when adrenalin is released continuously into the blood stream over a long period, as may happen during a busy day at the office, or in the anxious few days preceeding an examination, its effects may be less beneficial. Because the digestive system is "switched off" by adrenalin, we experience queasiness or indigestion, and if stress continues for too long, some of the so-called "businessman's diseases" like gastric ulcers may appear.

Thyroid disorders are quite common. In children, thyroid deficiency can cause stunted growth and low intelligence, but when it occurs in adults, a general sluggishness results. In some areas there is a lack of iodine in the diet, and the thyroid gland responds by growing to an enormous size. This causes a large swelling at the base of the neck, known as "goitre". Even a minute trace of iodine in the diet is sufficient to prevent this, so iodine is usually added to ordinary table salt in small amounts.

Diabetes

The best known glandular disorder is diabetes: an excess of glucose in the bloodstream caused by a poorly functioning pancreas. If untreated, this condition can lead to unconsciousness and death, but if the missing hormone, insulin, is replaced by frequent injections, the sufferer can lead a normal life.

▼ Pituitary overactivity produces giants with elongated limbs. The tiniest dwarves are produced when the pituitary fails to produce enough growth hormone.

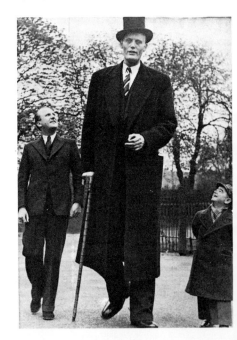

Reproducing mankind

One of mankind's highest functions is the drive to reproduce. The female body is extensively adapted to aid in conception of a child; to nourish it during pregnancy; to give birth without damaging the child; and to feed the child with milk after its birth. The major physical differences between man and woman reflect this need.

A woman has wider hips than a man, because the child has to pass through a gap in the rigid pelvis. In a woman, this gap is precisely the right size to allow the passage of a child. The different hip structure, and the need for specialised and bulky internal sex organs, means that the woman's abdomen is shaped rather differently from that of a man. Breasts are present in both men and women, but in a woman develop to full size under the influence of hormones in the bloodstream.

The advent of modern contraceptives has meant that reproduction need not be the natural consequence of intercourse. Contraceptive techniques are now available which give virtually certain protection from unwanted pregnancy, and some of these are much less obtrusive than older and less reliable methods. Several contraceptives rely on preventing the sperm from reaching the egg. The sheath or condom fits over the penis and stops the release of sperm into the vagina. The cap fits within the vagina and blocks the passage of sperms through the cervix. These mechanical methods are best used together with a chemical which kills any sperms getting past the contraceptive. The intra-uterine device (IUD) is a small plastic contraceptive fitted within the uterus, which prevents a fertilised egg from becoming implanted in the wall of the womb. The pill may operate in the same way by interfering with the body chemistry, or by stopping the release of eggs from the ovary.

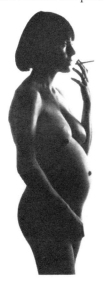

▲ The child within the womb is affected by its mother's dietary faults. Smoking can also have serious effects. Periodically campaigns are run to point out these dangers to pregnant mothers.

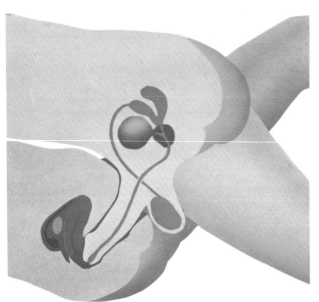

Sexual intercourse

During intercourse, the male penis is introduced into the vagina of the female partner, and is moved in a pumping action by rocking movements of the hips. Provided sufficient petting and foreplay has taken place, the vagina will be lubricated by liquid secreted from the mouth of the vagina and the vaginal walls. The sensations produced during intercourse on the glans of the penis and on the sensitive clitoris eventually result in orgasm for both partners, and a pool of semen is deposited at the entrance to the cervix.

The male organs

The testicles are suspended outside the body in a flexible bag; the scrotum. Within each testicle a tightly-coiled tubule produces sperms, which are stored in liquid produced in the seminal vesicles and prostate gland. At orgasm they are ejaculated along the urethra by a series of muscular contractions. Within the penis is tissue into which blood is forced during sexual arousal, causing it to become erect and ready for intercourse.

1 Seminal vesicles
2 Bladder
3 Prostate glands
4 Vas deferens
5 Urethra
6 Scrotum
7 Testicle
8 Seminiferous tubule
9 Foreskin
10 Glans

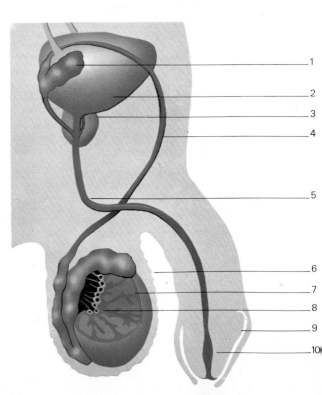

Conception

At monthly intervals, ripening egg cells are expelled from the ovary, and are passed down the Fallopian tube. Sperms introduced into the vagina during intercourse make their way through the mucus seal of the cervix and swim up the uterus where most perish. The survivors swim along the Fallopian tube to meet the egg, and a single sperm succeeds in fertilising it. The single cell divides into two, then into four, and continues dividing, doubling the number of cells each time. When it reaches the uterus $5\frac{1}{2}$ to 7 days after conception, the tiny ball of cells becomes attached to the thick endometrium, the womb lining. Here, as it continues to develop, it produces the placenta, a large and complex organ which acts as a "life support system". The placenta spreads into the mother's tissues, extracting nutrients and passing back the embryonic waste products, to be disposed of by the mother's bloodstream. Nos. 1—4 show fertilization; the fusion of the sperm and ovum nuclei. Nos. 5—8 show cell division, growth of placenta and attachment to the endometrium.

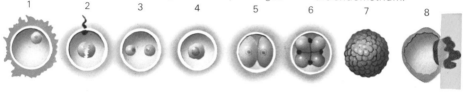

1   2   3   4   5   6   7   8

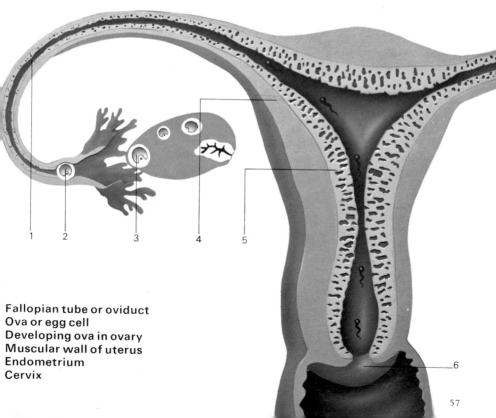

1   2   3   4   5

6

Fallopian tube or oviduct
Ova or egg cell
Developing ova in ovary
Muscular wall of uterus
Endometrium
Cervix

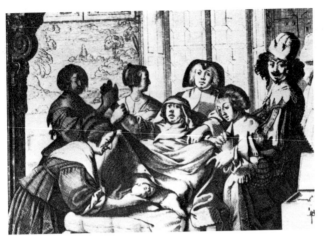

Sperm meets egg

By comparison with the female body, the sex organs of a man are relatively simple, consisting basically of two glands called testicles, which can produce about 200 million sperm cells each day. These are introduced into the woman during intercourse by means of the penis, which serves the dual function of reproduction and urination. Each tiny sperm contains half the blueprint for a human being: tiny threads called chromosomes which each contain many genes, each controlling a characteristic such as hair colour, height, and so on.

The other half of the blueprint is provided by the egg produced within the woman's ovaries. At birth, the ovaries of a female child already contain all the egg cells she will produce during her life. They become mature at roughly monthly intervals, and pass down the oviducts or Fallopian tubes, meeting the sperms introduced into the vagina during intercourse. Only a single sperm penetrates the egg cell, and in the act of fertilisation, completes the blueprint and triggers the growth of a new human being.

Conception

From the moment of fertilisation, or conception, growth of the embryo is swift. It grows on the wall of the uterus, first to a small blob of cells, then quickly developing into a tadpole-like creature with recognisable organs. During its early growth, the embryo passes swiftly through stages which we believe form part of our evolutionary past. Each of us, as embryo within our mother's womb, once resembled a fish, with gills, and then briefly possessed a circulatory system like that of an amphibian or reptile. Six weeks after conception we still had a tail, but by eight weeks, developed into a recognisable, tiny human being, about 25mm long, with distinguishable fingers and toes, all the vital organs of the body, and a working circulatory system.

From then on, to the moment of birth nine months after conception, the foetus increases steadily in size, feeding on nutrients extracted from the mother's bloodstream via the placenta, which is large sponge-like organ embedded in the wall of the uterus.

The placenta is the child's only lifeline

It is connected to the child by the thick tubular umbilical cord, through which it receives nutrients and oxygen, and disposes of waste material. At first, the body of the mother can easily cope with the tiny foetus growing within it. Morning sickness or nausea is very common, but usually passes off after a few weeks.

Demands on the mother

As the foetus continues to grow, it begins to make demands on the mineral reserves stored in the mother's body. Calcium is extracted from her bones and must be replaced by supplementing the diet with calcium-rich foods. Iron is removed from the mother's blood, and is transferred to the foetus to allow it to develop its own blood supply, so the mother may suffer slight anaemia.

The body of a pregnant woman is under a considerable physical strain during the latter part of her pregnancy. The increased weight she must carry causes uncomfortable changes in posture and makes sleeping difficult, and the heart and circulation also have to work much harder.

The birth

At full term, the child is ready to be born. Up until then, it has floated in a comfortable liquid-filled bag within the womb, sucking its thumb, and trying out limb movements which can be distinctly felt by the mother. When birth begins, its peace is interrupted by a violent and sometimes prolonged passage to the outside world. The powerful muscles of the uterus contract violently and spasmodically, while the cervix at the entrance to the womb dilates, allowing the baby to be forced down into the elastic tube of the vagina, and out through the vulva. This whole process can take as little as two hours in a woman who has previously given birth, or can be prolonged for many hours.

▼ The greatest effort during labour is delivery of the child's head. After this, the rest of the child follows quite easily.

▼ The final stage of labour is the delivery of the placenta, to which the baby is still attached by the umbilical cord.

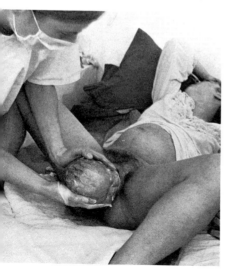
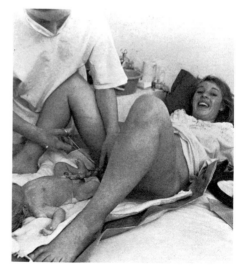

59

Age and ageing

Our cells have limited life spans, and human ageing is characterised by different groups of cells and organs becoming senile at different points in our lifetime.

Life and the cell

This is governed by the ability of cells to reproduce themselves. After the initial spurt of growth in youth, nerve cells do not reproduce. Any later damage to the nervous system is incompletely repaired, and as cells in the brain die off in extreme old age, there is a falling-off in mental

▼ In parts of the Ukraine and in mountainous areas in South America live many people claimed to be more than 150 years old, (although their age is doubted by some). Some of them ascribe their longevity to a diet of honey and nuts.

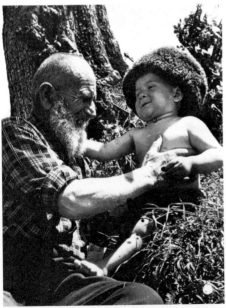

abilities; the onset of senility.

But long before this happens, the body has begun to decline. Most other body cells are capable of being renewed, but this capability deteriorates once we reach maturity. This is why children, whose cells can divide very rapidly, recover from wounds or sickness so much more quickly than adults. As the rate of cell renewal falls away in old age, bone fractures may never heal properly, and skin complaints like bed sores may cause problems.

The actual life span of the cell varies tremendously. White blood cells may live little more than a day, while bone cells survive for more than 25 years. The cells lining the intestine are shed at the rate of half a pound each day, and these are promptly redigested further down the gut.

Three score and ten

The inevitable end result of the ageing process is death, but the causes and time of death can vary enormously. The average life span of "three score years and ten" quoted in the Old Testament is almost exactly that of the average European or American. In developing countries, however, the average person may live only thirty to forty years, and a woman may be old at twenty-five.

In the aged, as the body begins to run down, so too does the immune system which normally protects us from disease and consequently more people die from the diseases of old age; the degenerative diseases. It is an unpleasant paradox that the longer we extend our lives, the more varied are the the diseases which will ultimately destroy us.

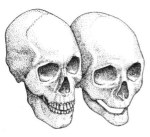

The ageing process

As cell replacement becomes less efficient, the inevitable processes of ageing become apparent. Different areas are affected at differing rates, and vary widely between individuals.

The changes affecting the head are most apparent. Greying hair (**1**) is obvious, but even the bones of the skull (**2**) shrink slightly. Cell loss has serious effects on the brain (**3**), and is the direct cause of senility. The eyes (**4**) lose their power to focus accurately, as the lense becomes harder. The ear-drums thicken, so hearing also becomes less efficient (**5**). Along with loss of the teeth with advancing age, the sense of taste deteriorates, so food becomes less appealing (**6**). Loss of cartilage shortens the spine (**7**), and the circulation may also begin to fail (**8**). Muscles (**9**) are not used so much, and tend to atrophy. Breast tissue (**10**) also atrophies after childbearing age. Elderly people tend not to eat proper meals, and suffer dietary deficiencies, while their stomachs

shrink in size (**11**). After the menopause, ovaries have little function, and become reduced in size (**12**), although the male sexual organs are little affected by advancing age. Joints stiffen (**13**) and bones become brittle (**14**), while the skin grows hard and wrinkled (**15**).

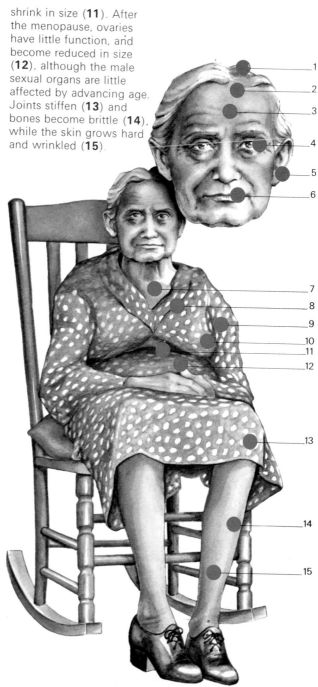

1
2
3
4
5
6
7
8
9
10
11
12
13
14
15

First aid

If someone has been injured, first *think*. If the casualty has severe injuries, sitting them up, or even giving them a drink could prove fatal. So the golden rule in first aid is, if in doubt—*don't*. However, most injuries are obviously minor, such as cuts, scratches and bruises, and can be safely treated at home. In addition, there are many minor disorders like headaches and colds which do not need professional medical attention. When a serious accident takes place in the home, it is usually better left untreated by the inexperienced. When medical aid can be summoned quickly, action is only necessary when the injuries threaten life.

The one accident situation where immediate action *must* be taken is when a person stops breathing. This might be the result of drowning, electrocution, suffocation, head injury caused by a fall, poisoning, or a variety of other accidents. If someone has stopped breathing, however, there may be a simpler cause—the breathing passages may be blocked by food, vomit, saliva, or even the tongue. This type of accident is particularly common in young children, and may happen when they vomit slightly during violent exercise. Whatever the cause, it is imperative that breathing is restarted quickly, as otherwise brain damage can result. Act quickly; lay the casualty flat on his back, and pull back the head while holding the jaws clenched. This prevents the tongue from falling back into the throat and blocking the air passages. If any foreign matter like sand or vomit can be seen in the victim's mouth or throat, scoop it out with the fingers.

▼ In an unconscious person the tongue may drop back into the throat, and prevent breathing.

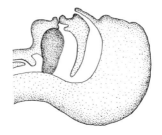

▼ Check that the tongue is not blocking the throat, and remove any foreign material.

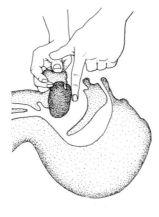

False teeth are a particular hazard, and often fall back into the throat of an unconscious person. If breathing does not start immediately, you must begin artificial respiration right away, by breathing directly into the casualty's lungs through the mouth or nose. In adults, the mouth-to-nose method is preferred, as it is less liable to make the casualty vomit. In children, however, it is more convenient to breathe into mouth and nose simultaneously. As you exhale deeply through the casualty's nose, it is necessary to hold their mouth firmly closed. If you are breathing into the mouth, however, pinch the nostrils to stop the escape of air. If the airways are not obstructed, you will see the chest of the casualty rise as you exhale. Remove your mouth, and the air will escape from the casualty's lungs. Each time you blow, turn your head to check that there is this regular rise and fall of the chest. This must be continued until breathing starts spontaneously, or in any event, for at least an hour. As soon as the casualty starts to respond you should see an improvement in his colour; usually after the first dozen or so inflations. When breathing starts, it will be weak and shallow, and will still need assisting. Time your breaths to coincide with those of the casualty, as his breathing gradually strengthens. When breathing has restarted, and can continue without help, the casualty will still be unconscious. He should be turned into the "unconscious position" shown below, preferably with the body slightly higher than the head, and watched carefully to make sure that breathing continues. Don't rush to get him to hospital; it is more important to make sure that breathing is strong, and will continue while the casualty is being moved.

► Tip the victim's head back, and make sure that nothing is clogging the airways. Blow into nose, or nose and mouth.

► Hold the casualty's mouth firmly closed while you blow into his nose; alternatively pinch the nose as you breathe into the mouth.

► Watch to make sure that the chest of the victim rises and falls as you breathe into him.

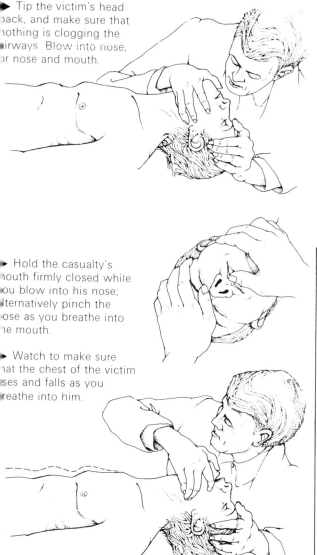

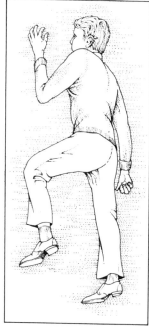

Self treatment

Commonsense should tell you whether or not a minor injury or disorder needs professional treatment. Head injuries and loss of consciousness, for instance, or deeply penetrating or infected wounds are potentially serious, and any home treatment would be inadequate and probably quite dangerous. Many minor problems can be successfully treated at home, however, and a well stocked emergency first aid kit should be a part of every household. Bandages, disinfectant, pins, plasters, scissors; most of the essentials are readily available.

Cuts and grazes

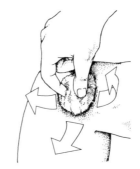

When the skin is broken, there are three objectives in treatment. Stop the bleeding; clean the wound; cover the wound while it heals.

Running water removes most dirt from the wound and wiping with cotton-wool *away* from the injury gets rid of surface dirt. A wash over with mild antiseptic helps prevent infection, but follow the directions on the bottle and don't apply the antiseptic at full strength. Bleeding should stop spontaneously if the wound is carefully cleaned and kept covered. When you cover with plaster or bandage, the wound may stick to the dressing, but petroleum jelly or a loose fitting dressing may prevent this.

Splinters

If you can remove a splinter with your fingers, or with

Burns

Any deep burn or blistered area bigger than about 30 mm (1¼ inch) across needs hospital treatment to avoid scarring. Smaller minor burns should be treated exactly like cuts and grazes, by careful cleaning and covering with a dressing. Aspirin helps reduce the pain.

Ultra-violet radiation in sunlight causes tanning of the skin, but before this protective colouring builds up, sunburn may be a problem. Calamine lotion eases the pain of minor sunburn,

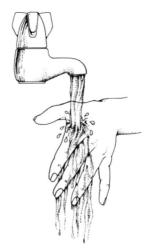

when the skin is only reddened. If a large area of skin has blistered, you will need medical attention, although for small areas, antihistamine cream may reduce the pain and inflammation. If someone is severely sunburned and is shivering or vomiting, it is possible that they have sun stroke; get medical assistance immediately. Chemical burns of the skin require specialised treatment, and washing with water is the only first aid which should be attempted.

weezers, no further treatment should be necessary, apart from cleaning the skin to avoid infection. However, infection can be introduced in the splinter, and if inflammation and swelling develops around the punc-

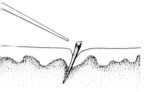

ure, medical treatment is advisable. If the splinter is broken off *level* with the skin, wash the area thoroughly and try to lift the splinter with a clean needle until it can be withdrawn. If it is *below* the skin surface, do not probe

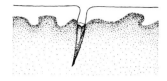

to try and locate it, or you will almost certainly cause infection—go to the doctor for proper treatment.

Digestion

There are innumerable freely available remedies for digestive upsets. Stomach pains, heartburn, diarrhoea, constipation, even haemorhoids, can all be self-treated effectively *in the short term*, with medicines available from any chemist. Take the pharmacist's advice by all means, but if the problem doesn't clear up within a few days, consult your doctor. Self-treatment can easily mask the symptoms of a more serious condition. It should never be necessary to take antacid powders, or laxatives continually as the underlying conditions usually result from a faulty diet.

Hangovers

There is *no* secret cure for a hangover, except time and patience. If you are hungover, the lining of your stomach will be red and inflamed, so taking aspirin will make matters worse. Drink plenty of water or milk, and the discomfort should ease fairly quickly. Normal headaches are best treated with ordinary aspirin.

Insect bites and stings

Treat insect bites, like sunburn, by applying calamine cream or lotion. Antihista-

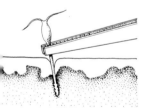

ine creams may reduce the swelling and itching of sting. If the sting is still in the wound, remove it with the finger nails or with tweezers, and wash the area thoroughly before applying calamine. If the swelling continues to develop, the sting may be infected, and will need medical treatment. When removing bee stings, be careful not to squeeze them, as you may press the poison sac attached to the skin, and inject more poison into the wound. Scratching always makes the itching worse.

Foreign bodies

Children are particularly prone to put stones, beads, etc., up their noses and in their ears, or more frequently, to swallow them. If you suspect that a child has put something up its nose, or in an ear, *don't* attempt to remove it—take the child to hospital. When

a foreign body is inhaled, it is usually immediately expelled by violent coughing. If not, place the casualty face down over a bed or table, with the head hanging over the edge. If the object is not speedily coughed up, get the casualty to hospital immediately. When a foreign body is swallowed, usually by a child, first find out what it was. Small objects like coins pass straight through the digestive tract, and reappear naturally within a week. If there is no evidence of them having been passed, seek medical advice.

Looking after your body

Looking after your body involves the exercise of commonsense, and an awareness of situations which hasten the natural decline of tissues with advancing years. It also means taking a long, cool look at many of the patent remedies and cosmetics which are advertised to slow down or reverse this process, but which can sometimes cause further damage.

Skin may seem delicate to the touch, but is in fact a fine form of leather, which is immensely strong and flexible. In ageing, the fibres supporting the skin become harder and more tightly packed, and the skin loses its elasticity. This is first apparent on the face and hands, where the skin is flexed a great deal. Rather than folding without leaving a trace, the skin of an older person creases permanently, causing lines. This unpleasant prospect is inevitable— no skin lotions or creams can halt its progress, or reverse its effects. Face packs and astringent lotions temporarily reduce wrinkles and "laughter lines", by shrinking and tightening the skin, but they cannot reach the deeper tissues where the hardening fibres are situated. For the adolescent, acne and greasy skin can cause severe embarrassment. Hormonal changes in the body chemistry cause these skin disorders, and there is little which can be done, other than meticulous washing to remove excess skin oil and minimise bacterial contamination. The condition usually disappears of its own accord as the body chemistry settles down. Overexposure to sun not only causes sunburn, but increases the natural ageing of the skin. There is no doubt that prolonged sun, wind and exposure to the elements causes reddening and roughness of the skin and this can be reduced by using creams which keep the skin moist and oily, particularly about the mouth and eyes. Avoiding skin exposure to powerful chemicals like bleach and detergent is only common sense.

Teeth

The illustration below shows the structure of teeth, and makes clear the problem of dental decay. Dental problems are largely a product of our evolutionary past. Our jaws have become so short that our teeth are crowded together, and so trap decaying food particles. Our mouths are ideal breeding grounds for bacteria, and these cause various problems. Acid produced by bacteria eats through

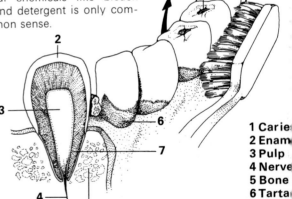

1 Caries
2 Enamel
3 Pulp
4 Nerve
5 Bone
6 Tartar
7 Dentine

the enamel and the dentine of the tooth until the soft pulp is exposed, and decay then proceeds in earnest. The only remedy is dental treatment, but much decay can be delayed or avoided by careful cleaning of the teeth. Brushing along the line of the teeth simply "skates over" the gaps between them—brushing up and down allows the bristles of the toothbrush to get in between them and remove the bacteria-laden plaque or film which develops on the tooth surface. To make a really thorough job of cleaning, use medicated dental floss between the teeth to remove plaque that even the most conscientious brushing cannot reach.

Tartar is a chalky, scale-like deposit which is formed on the teeth by saliva. If it is not periodically removed by a dentist it can damage the gums and allow bacteria to enter, where the teeth pass through the gums.

Fluoride additives in drinking water and toothpaste have been widely promoted to protect teeth against decay. There is evidence to show that in children, fluoride can reduce the amount of decay, but once the teeth have stopped growing, fluoride offers no protection. When fluoride has already been added to the drinking water, there is no extra benefit in using fluoride toothpastes, and too much fluoride can cause teeth to discolour.

Nails

Finger and toe nails are dead tissue, composed of the same material as hair. Ageing causes hardening and weakness of the nails with consequent painful splitting or cracking, but the nails are also useful indicators of other conditions. Poor diets often cause changes in the nails. Iron deficiency or anaemia may soften the nails and other illnesses can cause white specks which gradually pass up the nail and are trimmed off. Careful trimming of the nails reduces the tendency to splitting or cracking, but if they are cut too short, painful infections may result.

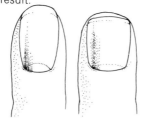

Nails should be trimmed to a squarish outline. If they are cut back at the sides into a true oval, the quick at the edges may be damaged.

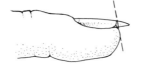

Unless there are cosmetic reasons for wanting long nails, they should be trimmed flush with the fleshy tip of the finger or toe.

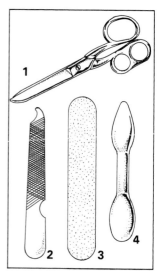

1 Use proper nail scissors for trimming. **2** and **3** Nail-file and sanding board reduce splitting.
4 You can improve nail shape by pushing back cuticles gently.

Hair

Care of hair is similar in many ways to that of the skin. Hair is a dead tissue, which is continuously produced from follicles in the scalp and other parts of the body. Sebaceous glands lubricate the hair shaft with an oil which provides a water-repellant coating. In neglected hair, this oil may build up to unacceptable levels, and must be removed by washing. But too frequent washing removes all the oil, making the hair dull and "lifeless". Sets and perms change the chemical structure of the hair, by heat or by chemical treatment, and unless this is expertly carried out, all the exposed part of the hair shafts may be damaged. Looking after normal hair means sensible washing and brushing, avoiding too much chemical treatment, and using hairdryers carefully so that the hair is not overheated. Greying is part of the natural ageing process, and like balding, cannot be treated or reversed. Dandruff is a condition where the tiny flakes of skin which are continually

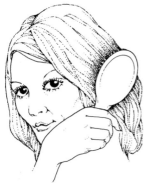

being shed from all over the body are retained on the scalp. This is caused by an oily skin, and frequent shampooing usually helps.

Eyes

Eyes are one of the most delicate parts of the body, and at the same time, among the best protected. It is very rarely that the eye is physically damaged by a foreign object as, if the object is large enough to be seen, the eye will blink shut before it can be touched. Obviously grit and dust can adhere to the eye, but the immediate

flow of tears will usually remove these particles. Rubbing the eyes will only result in painful scratches on the delicate cornea. Apart from using an eyebath to remove dirt, never attempt self-medication; go to the doctor or to hospital.

Feet

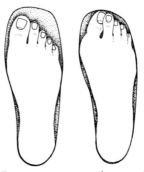

Feet are among the most easily damaged parts of the body, and damage caused by ill-fitting shoes can often be permanent. The foot is a

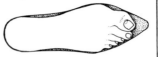

complex structure, and if the tiny bones it contains are forced out of position by pointed-toed shoes, or shoes which are too short, they may become permanently deformed and make walking extremely painful.

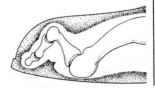

Exercising care

Like most other things, exercise is very good in moderation. The musculature of the human body differs from most other parts in that it is capable of developing to cope with increasing work, without suffering any damage. Muscle fibres divide and increase the actual size of the muscles when sufficient exercise is taken. Conversely, they become flabby and atrophy when too little exercise is taken. In excess, exercise can be very damaging, as the body which is not accustomed to heavy work takes several months to reach peak condition. Suddenly undertaking strenuous work without prior training can cause pulled muscles, slipped discs, and damaged joints — worse, in fact, than too little exercise. Treated sensibly, exercise can improve the overall health. It will minimise the circulatory diseases which usually occur in later life. Due to our fat-rich diet, a sticky substance called cholesterol accumulates in the bloodstream. This can become deposited on the walls of blood vessels, and causes hardening of the arteries in later life. Exercise keeps this dangerous substance circulating in the blood, and stops the damaging deposits from building up.

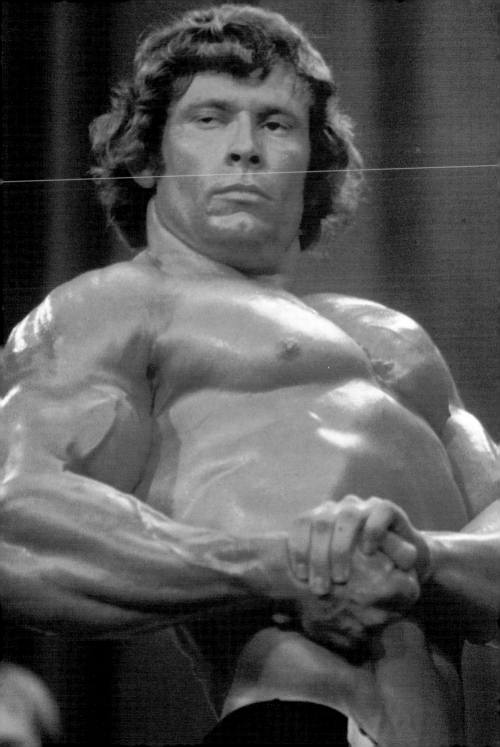

Exercises for muscle

Sensible exercising means building up over a number of weeks. Don't push yourself too much; if you feel tired you have probably had enough.

1 Press-ups Place the palms flat on the ground, beneath the shoulders. The whole body must be raised on the arms, without allowing the stomach to sag or the back to bend. Bend the arms until the chest lightly touches the floor, then straighten the arms to push the body back to the starting position.

2 Side bending Press the hands down alternate sides, bending at the waist. Eventually you should reach below the knees.

3 Half-squats Bend the knees to a semi-sitting position, while extending the arms horizontally. Return to the original position.

4 Sit-ups Lying on your back, rise to a semi-sitting position, until your hands reach your knees. Slowly return to original position.

5 Dorsal exercise Lying face down, clasp the hands behind the back, and raise trunk and legs from the ground.

6 Burpee Drop from the standing position into a crouch, with the palms on the floor. Shoot out the legs in the "press-up" position. Return to crouch and stand up.

7 Spot running Run on the spot for twenty "strides", then do a "half-squat".

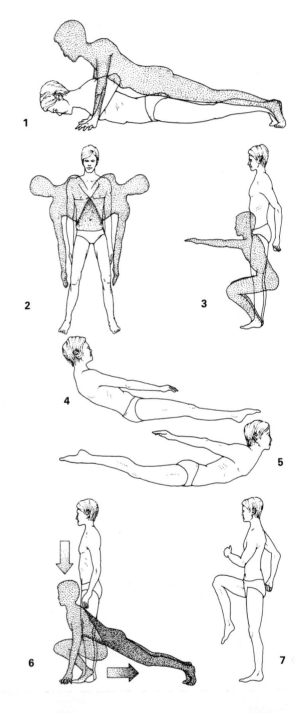

Exercises for weight

Exercise will not remove much weight, but is a useful way of toning up flabby muscles as you lose weight on a diet. Don't overdo it; just continue until you feel pleasantly tired.

When you find them easy, increase the number of times you do each exercise.

Jumps Raise your arms and jump, trying to reach an imaginary point well above your head. Repeat the jump several times.

2 Trunk raising Stand in a doorway, with your arms raised to touch the sides of the door frame above your head, and with your feet together. Now bend at the knees until you can rest your fingers on the floor, then return to the original position. Repeat several times.

3 Chair sits Sit across an ordinary armless chair, in a "sidesaddle" position. Place one hand on the chair back, then stand up and sit down 10 times, each time only barely touching the seat of the chair.

4 Supported press-ups Arrange yourself face-down across a chair, with your thighs supported and the flats of your hands on the floor. Bend your arms until your face touches the floor, then push back to the starting position. Do ten press-ups.

5 Leg lifts Sit on a chair, with your hands resting on the table. Now straighten your legs, and keeping them extended, raise them until they touch the underside of the table. Keep the back straight while raising legs.

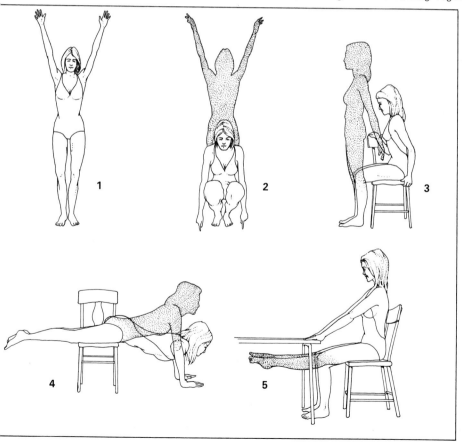

Can you trust your senses?

All of our senses are capable of being tricked, but of these none is so susceptible as vision. We rely on our eyes to interpret what we see in recognisable form, and even the simplest "view", requires a certain amount of interpretation. To all but the youngest child, a photograph is instantly recognisable, even if it is in black and white. But if a simple illustration or photograph is shown to a person who may previously have been blind for many years, or to one of the few remaining primitive people who have never seen pictures of any sort, then they are often unable to interpret it. Illusions, therefore, are often a result of preconceptions.

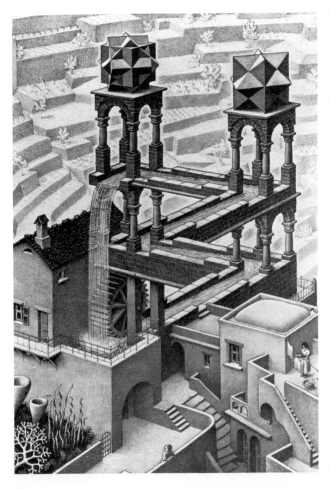

We interpret perspective according to rules which specify that objects nearest the eye are larger than those in the distance. This is purely a convention, however, which is not understood by some primitive people. We in turn think many of their artistic conventions are distorted or inaccurate.

Because we are continually making this mental effort to classify and interpret what we see, pictures which are deliberately designed to conflict with our convention are disturbing and may even be physically uncomfortable to look at. But our interpretations can be illuminating to the psychologist and give valuable insights into the working of damaged minds.

◄ "Waterfall" by Maurits Escher. This is an illusion of impossible perspectives. It defies the logic that water cannot flow uphill.

Colour blindness

This is a defect which is often inherited. Complete colour blindness is extremely rare, but between 4 and 8 percent of men and only 0.4 per cent of women are affected in varying degrees. Some people are ununable to distinguish the various shades of reds and greens, which presents problems at traffic signals. These people can manage quite well by relying on their ability to differentiate between intensities of light. Another symptom of colour blindness is being unable to see differences in shades of yellows and blues. The test card (right) shows the number 45 in shades of red.

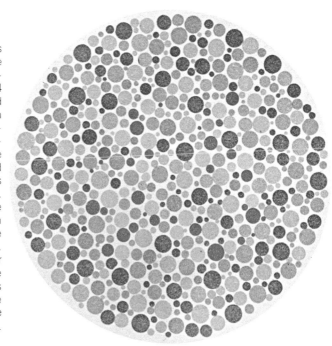

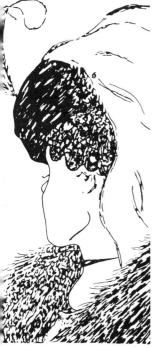

◀ This illusion involves seeing one of two familiar objects. We see either a young woman or an old woman with a shawl.

▼ If you stare at the flag until your eyes are tired and then look at a piece of white paper you should catch a glimpse of the Stars and Stripes in their true colours. This is called after image.

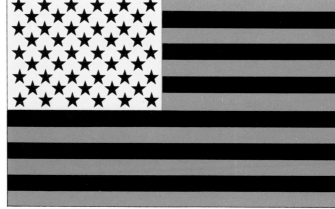

How emotional are you?

Everyone differs as to how much they are in control of their emotions and how much their emotions are in control of *them*. Medical science is appreciating more each day the importance this has to our mental and physical health. The balance is partly determined by temperamental factors—largely inherited, partly by training and partly by experience. This art lies in balancing recognition of the strength of one's emotion and exerting a reasonable degree of control. This questionnaire will help you to decide how the balance lies in your case.

1 If you could choose, would you prefer to work
   a In close contact with lots of people.
   b With a few people.
   c On your own.

2 Which statement is most true for you?
   a I think very little about other people's affairs.
   b I am interested in the lives of people I know well.
   c I am very interested in details of other people's lives and I enjoy hearing all the latest news.

3 When you greet your friends, do you
   a Nod, and say "Hello"
   b Smile, shake hands and say "Hello".
   c Give them a hug.

4 Would you consider writing to a Problem Page if you felt that you could not talk to your friends?
   a Certainly not.
   b Perhaps.
   c Yes.

5 You go into a coffee shop for a quiet cup of coffee, and find that the girl next to you is in tears. Would you
   a Want to say something comforting, but feel too shy.
   b Ask her if you can help.
   c Move your seat.

6 Someone you have just met says complimentary things about you and expresses a wish to know you better. Do you
   a Feel embarrassed.
   b View him with caution.
   c Feel flattered and disposed to like him.

7 When an important relationship in your life breaks up, do you
   a Feel bad, but go on as near to normal as possible.
   b Feel prostrated for at least a short time.
   c Shrug it off and block feeling of grief.

8 Do you
   a Ruthlessly throw away letters and mementos almost as soon as you get them.
   b Keep them for years.
   c Sort out such possessions every couple of years.

9 Do you suffer from feelings of guilt and remorse
   a Yes, even about events long over.
   b Occasionally.
   c No, you see no point in regrets.

10 At a particularly good performance at the theatre, do you
   a Applaud energetically.
   b Feel constrained about applauding.
   c Join in the applause, but feel rather silly.

11 You see someone you are pretty sure you recognise across the street.
   Would you
   a Walk on.
   b Cross over to say "Hello".
   c Wave, but if they don't respond walk on.

12 You hear a report that a friend has misunderstood an action of yours and is angry with you. Would you
   a Get in touch very soon to explain.
   b Leave them to work it out themselves.
   c Wait for a natural opportunity to get in touch, but say nothing about the misunderstanding.

13 What do you do with gifts you don't like?
   a Get rid of them fast.

b Keep them lovingly.

c Hide them and bring them out only when the giver comes to see you.

4 Do demonstrations, rituals or patriotic occasions

   a Leave you cold.

   b Move you to tears.

   c Embarrass you.

5 Which statement is most true for you?

   a I am wary about trusting my feelings.

   b My feelings are my main guide in my actions.

   c Feelings do not matter —consequences do.

▸CORES

1	a 3	b 2	c 1
2	a 1	b 2	c 3
3	a 1	b 2	c 3
4	a 1	b 2	c 3
5	a 2	b 3	c 1
6	a 2	b 1	c 3
7	a 2	b 3	c 1
8	a 1	b 3	c 2
9	a 3	b 2	c 1
0	a 3	b 1	c 2
1	a 1	b 3	c 2
2	a 3	b 1	c 2
3	a 1	b 3	c 2
4	a 1	b 3	c 2
5	a 2	b 3	c 1

om a questionnaire of this nd it is impossible to go to very fine detail and for is reason scores are classi-ed into three groups, which e could term Cerebral pes (score between 15 d 25), Balanced types core between 26 and 35), d Emotive types (score tween 36 and 45).

You will find yourself with a score lying somewhere between 15 and 45. Check your score against the vertical scale to get a rough idea of your rating, and then look at the more detailed analysis below for a deeper discussion.

45 Explosively emotional— could be alarming to self and others.

40 Highly emotional—and other people are aware of it!

35 Expresses emotions freely — but not unwisely.

30 Sometimes freely emotive—sometimes repressed.

25 Finds difficulty in expressing emotions.

20 Always seems in control —may resent emotion in others.

15 Apparently completely unemotional — probably repressively so.

ANALYSIS

The Cerebral Type

If you scored in this group you are basically of the type known as "cool, calm and collected". You rarely get excited about anything (or you rarely *seem* to) and even the most difficult or demanding situation never seems to push you into violent action. Even if you do get angry you tend to do so in a controlled and "seething" way. Your main weakness is that you will be unresponsive to or, if your score is very low, perhaps *incapable* of accepting emotion in others.

Balanced Type

This is an average score. You are a person who, in common with the bulk of mankind, tends to find periods when you seem to be kept pretty well under control. Even in the worst circumstances, if you really grit your teeth, you can stop yourself flying off the handle. It is very unlikely that you have ever had a really big row with anybody—domestic tiffs not included.

Emotive Type

There is no doubt about it, you are highly emotional with a very strong tendency for emotions to get the better of you. Many is the time you will have said to yourself "Why *did* I do that" or "How could I have said such a thing?" If you are a woman, you are a ready prey to tears and scenes. If you are a man, you will be aggressive and dominant, inclined to shout a bit and throw your weight around.

Eating the right way

Food is, quite literally, fuel for the body. It is "burned" to produce the energy which powers the human machine, the raw materials for growth, and replacement tissues when these are required.

Our diet consists of three basic components: protein, fat, and carbohydrate. These are taken into the body as food, and broken down by digestion into simple substances which can be absorbed into the body and used as fuel, or as building material.

In practice, of course, people living in the developed nations consume very much more than they need, especially of energy foods. The excess must be accounted for, and is usually converted into fat—the body's way of storing food.

Carbohydrates

Much of our food intake is in the form of carbohydrates,

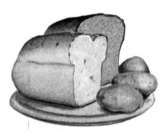

either as starch, in potatoes, bread, etc., or as sugar. Carbohydrates are excellent sources of energy, but contain little of the nutrient material needed to build up tissues.

Consequently, the huge amounts of excess carbohydrate in our diets is largely converted to fat, and carbohydrates are the easiest food to cut out or reduce when attempting to lose weight.

Protein

In most of the developed nations, the daily protein intake is about 110g daily. The generally recommended minimum protein requirement is about 70g per day, so we consume considerably more protein than we actually need.

Protein is the basic material used for building our own tissues, and is converted on digestion into amino acids. Children need adequate dietary protein for growth, and are the first to suffer protein deficiency in countries where famine is common.

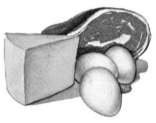

Fat

Fat provides the body with a large amount of energy in a very concentrated form. We consume fat and protein in about equal proportions, most coming from meat, with a smaller quantity in our vegetable food. Animal fats are often blamed for causing increased cholesterol levels

in the blood. Excess cholesterol contributes towards heart disease and hardening of the arteries. For this reason, those who are known to be suffering from such cardiovascular diseases should avoid animal fats.

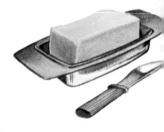

Vitamins

Vitamins, rather like hormones, have potent effects on the body in minute quantities. they are indispensable to life, yet in most cases cannot be manufactured in the body, and must be obtained from the diet. It is unlikely that many would suffer from serious vitamin deficiency today, yet vitamin tablets are sold in vast quantities throughout the world, and are consumed quite indiscriminately. There are about forty known vitamins, but those listed below are most commonly available.

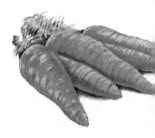

Vitamin A: deficiency can cause poor night vision, increased susceptibility to infection, and poor skin condition. It is normally present in large quantities in liver, rose-hips, butter, and carrots.

Vitamin B: there are three main B group vitamins: B_1 (Thiamine), Riboflavin and Niacin (Nicotinic Acid), and they are among the most potent chemicals in their effects in the body. Among

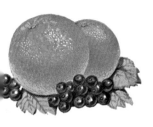

other B group vitamins are B_6, Folic Acid and B_{12}. Deficiencies cause a whole range of very serious diseases, now fortunately very rare, such as pellagra, and beri-beri.

Vitamin C: nearly all fruit contains large amounts of Vitamin C, which prevents scurvy. Most Vitamin C is destroyed during cooking, so it is important to eat fresh fruit. Recently advocated for prevention of colds.

Vitamin D: deficiency causes rickets, a serious bone deformity. Sources of this vitamin are fish oils, and exposure to sunlight, but recently it has been demonstrated that too much Vitamin D can have ill effects.

Vitamin E: although many extravagant claims have been made for this vitamin, none have been upheld, and there is no clear understanding of its normal function in humans.

Vitamin K: we obtain this vitamin in our diet, and from bacteria living in the digestive system. It plays an essential part in causing blood clotting, but is only needed in minute quantities, so there is little point in taking excessive amounts.

Minerals

Over a dozen minerals are essential to us, the most important being calcium, iron and iodine. Others include sodium, potassium, chloride, magnesium, phosphorus, fluoride and tiny amounts of elements such as copper. Many of these minerals are found in water.

Calcium: milk and cheese are the richest sources of this mineral, which is needed to maintain the skeleton and teeth.

Iron: present in the red blood pigment haemoglobin and is involved in the transfer of oxygen to the tissues; inadequate intake causes anaemia.

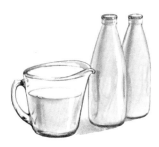

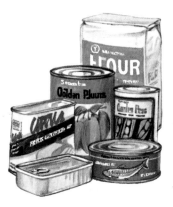

Iodine: deficiency causes goitre, and in areas of the world where intake from water is low, iodine is added to foodstuffs, particularly salt.

A healthy diet

Although in developed countries intakes of all necessary nutrients are usually above minimum levels, with a result that many suffer from such problems as overweight, some people's diets are dangerously low in such nutrients as iron and the B vitamins. Women during pregnancy require greater amounts of all nutrients, which in the case of calcium and Vitamin C, should be double the usual minimum. Moreover in our usually over-abundant diet, we are also taking in a variety of substances which our bodies are not equipped to handle.

Every time we eat tinned or ready-prepared food, we consume varying quantities of preservatives, and a range of artificial flavourings and colouring agents. It is difficult to determine the long-term effect of these substances on the body, and many feel it wiser to avoid them as far as possible, by eating fresh foods.

Nutrition tables

Table I gives the daily amount necessary, for various age-groups, of the major nutritional requirements. Values are a little above the absolute minimum necessary, but give a level for normal life. Energy is given in kilocalories (the "calorie"), protein in grams and all the others in milligrams except for Vitamin A which is in International Units (iu's) to simplify its complex origins.

Table II gives further information about the nutrients covered in the first table. For a variety of common foods three values are given **A, B** and **C.**
A is the amount of a particular nutrient in 100 grams of the given food.
B is the percentage of daily requirements for a man aged 19–35 who is moderately active provided by 100 grams of each food.

C performs the same task for an average teenage girl. All values are necessarily rounded but they do serve to give a good rough guide.
Figures in Table I are from the DHSS pamphlet *Recommended Intakes of Nutrients for the United Kingdom,* and the nutrient values for foods in Table II are from a bulletin of the United States Department of Agriculture.

Table II—Nutrients contained in 100 grams of various foods.   (— indicates a very small am

Food & Quantity	Energy			Protein			Calcium			Iron	
	A	B	C	A	B	C	A	B	C	A	B
	kcal	%	%	gm	%	%	mg	%	%	mg	%
Milk—half a cup	66	2	3	3.7	5	6	118	24	17	0.04	$\frac{1}{2}$
Cheddar cheese—3½ ozs	410	14	18	25.0	33	43	760	152	100	1.1	11
Eggs—2 large	160	5	7	12.0	16	20	54	11	8	2.2	22
Bread—white, 3 slices	270	9	12	8.6	11	15	84	17	12	0.7	7
Bread—"w'meal" 3 slices	241	8	10	9.0	12	16	84	17	12	3.0	30
Beef—sirloin steak, grilled	388	13	17	23.5	31	41	10.6	2	1	2.9	29
Liver—calves	228	7	10	26.3	35	45	10.5	2	1	8.8	88
Haddock—fried in crumbs	165	6	7	20.0	27	34	40	8	6	1.18	12
Sardines—4 average size	206	7	9	23.5	31	41	438	88	62	2.9	29
Fish fingers—4½	176	6	8	16.7	22	29	11	2	1	0.4	4
Cabbage—average portion	21	1	1	1.38	2	2	44	9	6	0.28	3
Carrots—2 average, cooked	31	1	1	0.6	1	1	33	7	5	0.6	6
Peas—a good portion	72	2	3	5.6	8	10	23	5	3	1.8	18
Potatoes—1 medium	66	2	3	1.6	2	3	5.7	1	1	0.5	5
Apples—one small apple	47	2	3	—	—	—	5.3	1	1	0.27	3
Orange juice—½ a cup	45	1	2	0.8	1	1	11	2	1	0.2	2
Peanuts—2 small packets	580	19	25	26.0	35	45	74	15	11	2.1	21
Cornflakes—4 portions	400	13	17	8.0	11	14	16	3	2	1.6	16
Beer—½ a cup	42	1	2	0.27	$\frac{1}{2}$	$\frac{1}{2}$	5	1	1	—	—
Ice cream—one portion	192	6	8	4.5	6	8	146	29	21	0.08	1
Milk chocolate—3½ ozs	518	17	23	7.1	9	12	232	46	33	1.1	11
Spinach—one good portion	22	1	1	2.8	4	5	93	18	13	2.2	22

Table I—Daily requirements of major nutrients for a healthy life.

Age/Sex Group	Energy kcal	Protein gms	Calcium mg	Iron mg	Vitamin A IU's	Vitamin B_1 mg	Riboflavin mg	Niacin mg	Vitamin C mg
Boys/ Girls 0–9 years	800–2,100	20–53	600	6–10	4,500	0.3–0.8	0.4–1.0	5–11	15–20
Boys 10–18 years	2,500–3,000	63–75	700	13–15	5,750–7,500	1.0–1.2	1.2–1.7	14–19	25–30
Girls 10–18 years	2,300	58	,,	,,	,,	0.9	1.2–1.4	13–16	25
Men 19–35 av. activity	3,000	75	500	10	7,500	1.2	1.7	18	30
Men 36–65 av. activity	2,900	73	,,	,,	,,	,,	,,	,,	,,
Men 66+	2,300	59	,,	,,	,,	0.9	,,	,,	,,
Women 19–55	2,200	55	,,	12	,,	,,	1.3	15	,,
Women 56+	2,000	51	,,	10	,,	0.8	,,	,,	,,
Women, preg., lactating	2,400, 2,700	60, 68	1,200	15	12,000	1.0, 1.1	1.6, 1.8	18, 21	60

Vitamin A			**Vitamin B_1**			**Riboflavin**			**Niacin**			**Vitamin C**		
A	B	C	A	B	C	A	B	C	A	B	C	A	B	C
IU's	%	%	mg	%	%	mg	%	%	mg	%	%	mg	%	%
143	2	2	0.03	2	3	0.17	10	13	0.08	½	½	0.8	3	3
1,320	17	20	0.035	3	3½	0.46	27	35	—	—	—	0	0	0
1,180	15.6	18	0.1	8	10	0.30	13	23	—	—	—	0	0	0
—	—	—	0.07	6	7	0.09	5	7	1.1	6	7	—	—	—
—	—	—	0.3	25	30	0.01	½	¾	2.8	15½	18½	—	—	—
59	1	1	0.06	5	6	0.19	11	14½	4.7	26	31	—	—	—
3,100	708	817	0.085	7	8½	4.16	245	320	16.5	92	110	26.3	88	105
—	—	—	0.035	3	3½	0.07	4	5	3.18	18	21	2.35	8	9½
224	3	3½	0.02	2	2	0.20	12	15	5.4	30	36	—	—	—
—	—	—	0.04	3	4	0.07	4	5	1.59	9	10½	—	—	—
131	2	2	0.04	3	4	0.04	2	3	0.28	2	2	33.0	110	132
0,500	140	162	0.054	5	5½	0.05	3	3½	0.48	3	3	6.0	20	24
540	7	8	0.28	23	28	0.11	6	8	2.3	13	15	21.0	69	84
—	—	—	0.09	8	9	0.03	2	2¼	1.15	6	7½	16.4	55	66
33	½	½	0.05	5	5	0.03	2	2¼	0.13	1	1	4.0	13	16
203	3	3	0.09	8	9	0.03	2	2¼	0.4	2	2½	50.3	170	201
—	—	—	0.3	25	30	0.13	7½	10	17.0	94	113	0	0	0
0	0	0	0.44	37	44	0.08	5	6	2.0	11	13	0	0	0
—	—	—	0.03	2½	3	0.03	2	2¼	0.6	3	4	—	—	—
444	6	7	0.038	3	4	0.21	12	16	0.08	½	½	0.75	2½	3
286	4	4½	0.07	6	7	0.36	21	28	0.36	2	2½	—	—	—
,100	108	125	0.07	6	7	0.14	8	11	0.56	3	4	27.8	93	111

Food of nations

Calories consumed per person each day in different parts of the world

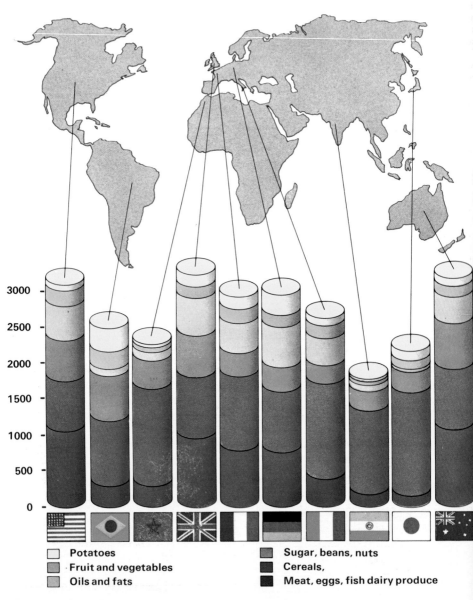

Potatoes

Fruit and vegetables

Oils and fats

Sugar, beans, nuts

Cereals,

Meat, eggs, fish dairy produce

Life Expectancy at Birth

hese figures give the average between male
nd female life expectancy at birth. The female
gure is always higher, often by as much as
ve years. Figures are necessarily approximations.
o world standards exist for the actual
ollection of data, and records in different
ountries may be completed at different times.
urther information can be found in the *United
ations' Statistical Yearbook* which is published
early and available in most reference libraries.

Life Expectancy at Birth

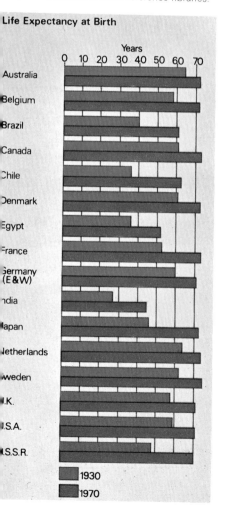

Causes of death

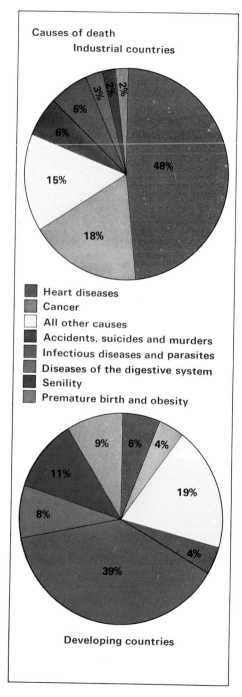

Industrial countries

- Heart diseases
- Cancer
- All other causes
- Accidents, suicides and murders
- Infectious diseases and parasites
- Diseases of the digestive system
- Senility
- Premature birth and obesity

Developing countries

The skeleton

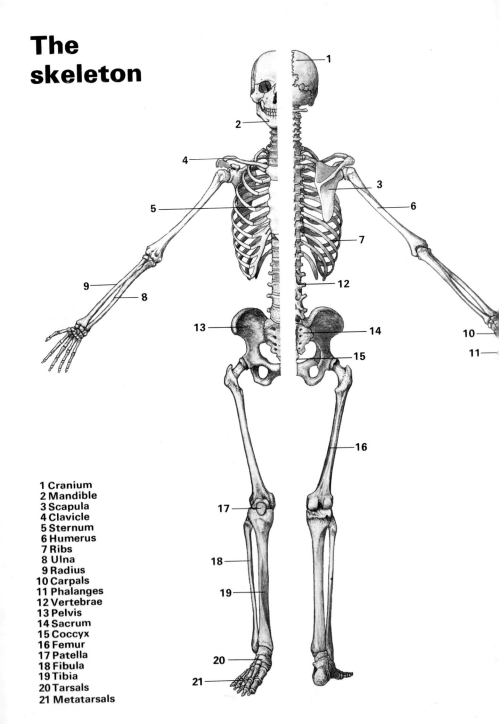

1 Cranium
2 Mandible
3 Scapula
4 Clavicle
5 Sternum
6 Humerus
7 Ribs
8 Ulna
9 Radius
10 Carpals
11 Phalanges
12 Vertebrae
13 Pelvis
14 Sacrum
15 Coccyx
16 Femur
17 Patella
18 Fibula
19 Tibia
20 Tarsals
21 Metatarsals

The muscles

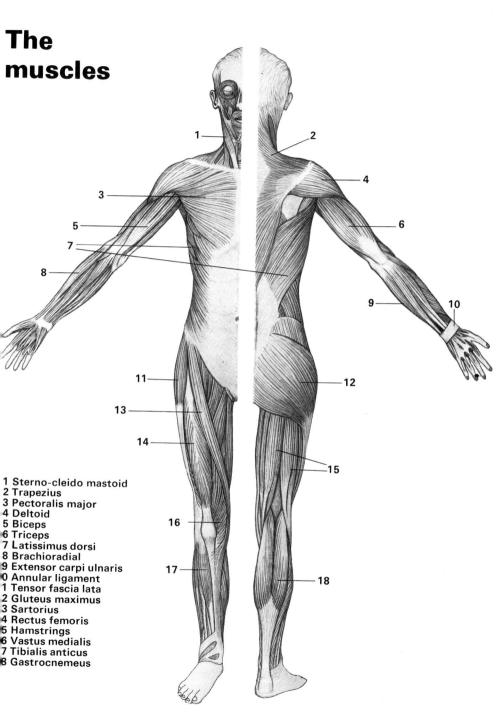

1 Sterno-cleido mastoid
2 Trapezius
3 Pectoralis major
4 Deltoid
5 Biceps
6 Triceps
7 Latissimus dorsi
8 Brachioradial
9 Extensor carpi ulnaris
0 Annular ligament
1 Tensor fascia lata
2 Gluteus maximus
3 Sartorius
4 Rectus femoris
5 Hamstrings
6 Vastus medialis
7 Tibialis anticus
8 Gastrocnemeus

The circulation

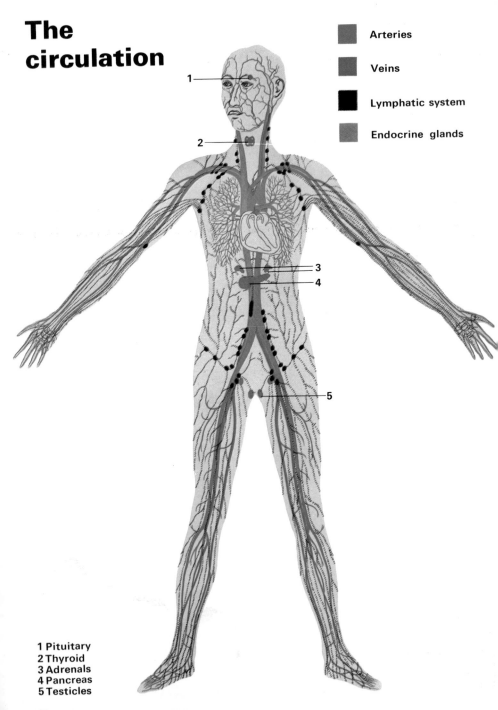

Arteries

Veins

Lymphatic system

Endocrine glands

1 Pituitary
2 Thyroid
3 Adrenals
4 Pancreas
5 Testicles

The vital organs

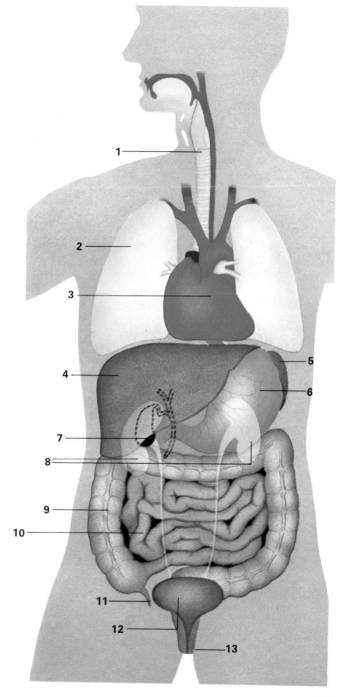

1 Trachea
2 Lungs
3 Heart
4 Liver
5 Spleen
6 Stomach
7 Gall bladder
8 Kidney
9 Colon
10 Small intestine
11 Appendix
12 Bladder
13 Rectum

The nervous system

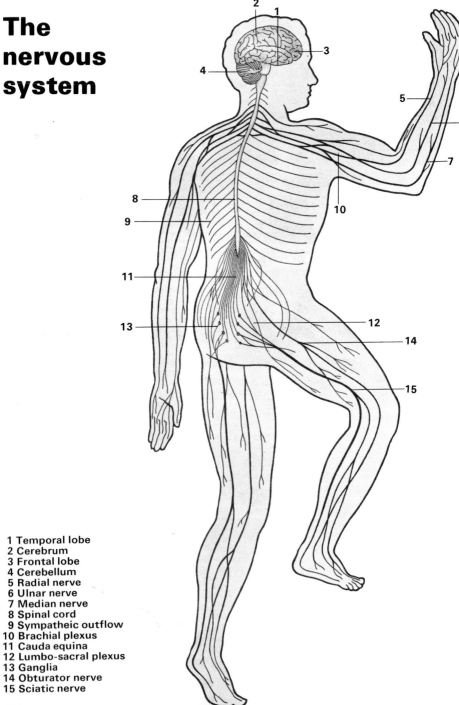

1 Temporal lobe
2 Cerebrum
3 Frontal lobe
4 Cerebellum
5 Radial nerve
6 Ulnar nerve
7 Median nerve
8 Spinal cord
9 Sympatheic outflow
10 Brachial plexus
11 Cauda equina
12 Lumbo-sacral plexus
13 Ganglia
14 Obturator nerve
15 Sciatic nerve

How do you measure up?

Average weight targets are shown in bold

All weights without clothes

Men
dd 3 kg for clothes
dd 25 mm for shoes

Women
dd 2½ kg for clothes
dd 50 mm for shoes

b=0.45kg

kg=9st 6lb
)kg=11st
)kg=12st 8lb
)kg=14st 2lb

height without shoes	suitable weight range		fat range		very fat range	
metres	kg	kg	kg		kg	
Men						
1.550	47½	**53**	58	to	63½	and over
1.575	49	**54½**	60	to	65½	and over
1.600	50½	**55¾**	61¼	to	67	and over
1.625	51¼	**57**	63	to	68¼	and over
1.650	53	**59**	64½	to	70¼	and over
1.675	54½	**60¾**	66¾	to	72½	and over
1.700	56¼	**62½**	69	to	75¼	and over
1.725	58	**64½**	70¾	to	77	and over
1.750	59½	**66¼**	73	to	79½	and over
1.775	61¼	**68½**	75¼	to	82	and over
1.800	63½	**70¼**	77½	to	84½	and over
1.825	65½	**72½**	79½	to	86¾	and over
1.850	67	**74½**	81¾	to	89½	and over
1.875	69	**76½**	84½	to	92	and over
1.900	71¼	**79**	86¾	to	94¾	and over
Women						
1.425	39½	**44**	48	to	52½	and over
1.450	40¼	**45**	49½	to	54	and over
1.475	41¾	**46½**	51	to	55¼	and over
1.500	43	**47½**	52½	to	57	and over
1.525	44	**49**	54	to	59	and over
1.550	45¼	**50¼**	55¼	to	60¼	and over
1.575	46¾	**52**	57	to	62	and over
1.600	48	**53½**	59	to	64½	and over
1.625	50	**55¾**	61¼	to	66¾	and over
1.650	51¾	**57½**	63	to	69	and over
1.675	53	**59½**	65¼	to	71¼	and over
1.700	55	**61¼**	67	to	73	and over
1.725	56¾	**63**	69	to	75½	and over
1.750	58	**65**	71¼	to	77½	and over
1.775	60	**66¾**	73	to	80	and over

ased on a table in the *Which? Slimming Guide* with the permission of the Consumers' Association.

Book list

to the brain when we are asleep? How does memory work? How does psychiatric treatment affect the brain? This book contains all this and more, and must be the clearest description yet of a very complicated subject.

The Penguin Medical Encyclopedia, Peter Wingate, Penguin Books, 1972, £1.50.
This indispensible little book contains everything most people will want to know about the body, in sickness and in health. It provides a straightforward "translation" of medical terms in layman's language, and is well cross-referenced to allow the reader to follow up related subjects in detail.

A Textbook of Human Biology, J. K. Inglis, Pergamon Press, 1974 £3.75, paperback £1.95.
A basic textbook of human biology, intended for the student. This book is a mine of information, but is intended as a reference, rather than for easy reading.

Man Alive: A Study of Human Physiology, G. L. McCulloch, Aldus Books, 1967.
Well-illustrated book which describes the working of the various systems of the body, rather than their structure.

Manipulation: Is Your Brain Your Own? E. Lausch, Fontana 1975 (Aidan Ellis 1974). £4.50.
A fascinating guide through the complexities of the human brain. The working of the "normal" brain is described in everyday language, and the effects of drugs on the brain is considered. What happens

The Pleasure Areas, H. J. Campbell, Eyre Methuen, 1973. £0.95.
How the brain determines our behaviour. *The Pleasure Areas* explores the mechanisms of the brain, and relates them to normal and abnormal behaviour patterns. It provides a link between the neurology or structure of the human brain, and the psychology of the mind.

An Introduction to the Study of Man, J. Z. Young, Oxford University Press, 1971, £9.00, paperback £3.95.
Professor Young's book is the most comprehensive survey of man and his body available in a single book. It covers the complete spectrum, from evolution to ageing, in a way which is scientifically impeccable, but easily assimilated by the layman. There is no better source book.

Body Time, G. G. Luce, Paladin, 1973 (Maurice Temple Smith, 1972), £1.25.
The biological clocks within our bodies control our physical functions, forcing them into regular cycles. They also have drastic effects on our moods and emotions. This book explains how they operate, and shows how the "off-days" we all experience can arise.

The Fluoride Question, A. L. Gotsche, Davis-Poynter, 1975, £4.00.
Whether we like it or not, most of us are forced to drink fluoridated water. Fluoride is added by the water authorities to protect children's teeth against decay. But is it safe? And does it work? *The Fluoride Question* discusses the arguments for and against fluoridation, and concludes that the case is "not proven"

Body and Drug, Ed. M. Jefferies, Sociopack, 1973.
A pack containing a series of cards which describe the systems of the body, and discuss the disorders which affect them, and the drugs which are used in these disorders. They explain why a particular drug is used, and how it can affect the body.

Man and Food, Magnus Pyke, World University Library, 1970. £0.80.
Magnus Pyke is a distinguished nutritional scientist and in this book he gives an authoritative review of what we eat, and how it affects us. If you want to know the nutritional values of all our basic foods, you will find them here, in easily digestible form. The relative merits of fresh, canned, and frozen foods are considered, and a number of myths exploded. This book is essential reading for food faddists or gluttonous eaters.

The Magic of the Senses, V. B. Droscher, Panther, 1971 (W. H. Allen, 1969). £0.50.
We take our senses for granted and are only dimly aware of their potentialities. This book shows how our senses work, and how restricted is our

awareness of our environment, compared with the vastly more efficient senses of animals. Complicated sensory mechanisms are simply described, in a very readable account.

The Puzzle of Pain,
R. Melzac, Penguin, 1973, 90p.
Nagging pains can be bothersome for days, but in the heat of battle serious injuries may not even be noticed. Professor Melzack explains what pain is, and how it can be alleviated.

Fads and Fallacies in the Name of Science,
M. Gardner, Dover Publications, £2.50.
Martin Gardner unerringly singles out many pseudo-scientific movements, and explodes their wilder theories. If you want to know the scientific basis for homeopathic medicine, osteopathic manipulation, and health foods like yogurt, wheat germ, and yeast, this is the book to consult. But be prepared to find your own pet theories ruthlessly demolished.

A Dictionary of Symptoms,
J. Gomez, Paladin, 1970, £1.75.
Self-diagnosis is a sure way to antagonise your doctor. Hypochondriacs should use this book with discretion.

Family Health,
Good Housekeeping Family Library, Sphere Books Ltd., 1975. £0.95.
A practical guide to looking after the family, in a crisis, and in day-to-day situations.

Pure, White and Deadly,
J. Yudkin, Davis-Poynter, 1972. £1.50.
If you are trying to cut down on your sugar intake, Professor Yudkin's book should give you added incentive. Sugar is implicated in diabetes, coronary thrombosis, tooth decay, and a host of other diseases.

Photographic Anatomy of the Human Body, C. Yokochi,
University Park Press, 1971 £6.75.
No diagram or drawing can do justice to the complexities of the human body. For those with strong stomachs, this book illustrates our intricate structure in detail, by photographs of actual dissections.

Consumers' Association Publications:
Eyes Right £1.25.
Caring for Teeth £1.25.
Care of the Feet £1.50.
Health for Old Age £1.50.
Which Way to Slim? £3.95.
Sex With Health £1.75.
These series of informative booklets have a direct no-nonsense approach, giving all the basic information about each subject. The last two on the list are particularly recommended.

Behold Man, Lennert Nilsson, Harrap, 1974, £15.00.
An expensive but lavishly illustrated book covering the human frame in detail.

Time-Life Science Library:

The Body, A. E. Nourse, 1971, £5.50.
An examination of how the body is constructed and how it functions backed up by considerable illustration.

The Mind, J. R. Wilson, 1971, £5.50.
The same highly illustrated approach describing the nervous system and summarising the most recent research into such subjects as learning, intelligence and mental illness.

Growth, J. M. Tanner and G. R. Taylor, 1966, £5.50.
Text and pictures trace the time-table of human development from conception to maturity, describing the many patterns which growth displays and exploring the frontiers of new research which may enable man to influence his own growth.

Food and Nutrition,
W. H. Sebrell and J. J. Haggerty, 1972, £5.50.
Explains how man finds his food, gives a clear, detailed account of the processes of nutrition, by which the body breaks food down to essential nutrients, examines the fads and fancies which have influenced man's choice of foods throughout history, and draws sober conclusions about the state of the world's food supplies in an era of rapid population growth.

The Human Body, Isaac Asimov, Signet Books, £1.25.
This chatty and informative study of the human anatomy and physiology is written in layman's language and yet goes into great detail and is thoroughly absorbing.

General infor- mation

Vocational Courses

Much information about the human body from a biological standpoint is covered by examination courses (mainly GCE) in "Biology" or more specifically in "Human Biology". Some examination boards also offer such subjects as "Nutrition", although this subject will often be included under an umbrella such as "Home Economics".

Moving on to further education, the medical profession is the obvious place to pursue an interest in the human body. Training is long and arduous and anyone who seeks further specialisation beyond the qualification to become a GP will take even longer.

It is possible to study nutrition at a higher level, though courses are not plentiful and study is naturally of a highly technical nature. With an enormous world population to feed, specialists in this subject have an important rôle to play.

Information about all courses can be obtained from local colleges, or in the case of university and medical colleges, from the **Universities Central Council on Admissions (UCCA)**, PO Box 28, Cheltenham, Gloucestershire, GL50 1HY, Tel: Cheltenham (0242) 59091, who will supply lists of courses available.

Recreational Courses

There is a wide range of courses available which have direct relevance to the healthy human body. Enquiries at the local "evening" college will very likely produce information on "keep fit" courses (often divided between different age groups), courses in yoga and related subjects and often courses related to cookery, on eating a balanced diet. In large urban areas courses may be found on a greater range of subjects and it is always worth enquiring at the local college or town hall, or if in London consulting the publication *Floodlight* which covers all non-vocational courses in the ILEA area.

Private clubs can often be used for courses in weight loss or keeping fit, these will be found in the Yellow Pages under "Health Clubs". Courses at these clubs will tend to be expensive.

Sports

Apart from the private health clubs mentioned above, those who want to keep their bodies fairly fit have ample recreational opportunities even in large urban areas. There are swimming baths, tennis courts, sports fields, and sometimes large sports complexes in many areas which are open to the public at no more than a small charge, and full information can be obtained from local town halls.

Medical Help

The first step if you need medical help of any kind is your family doctor, or if you don't have one, the Out Patients department of the local hospital. Whether you need medical treatment, psychiatric help, or just advice, your GP will help you or direct you to someone else who is better equipped to do so. If you have problems which you may not want to approach a GP about, the following contacts may be useful:

The Samaritans, 01-626 9000 in London, or look in the phone book; will always give you a sympathetic ear.

Release, l Elgin Avenue, London W9. 01-603 8654 will help you with a variety of problems including drugs.

Family Planning Association, 27 Mortimer Street, London W1A 4OW. 01-636 7866, for all reproduction problems. They can also help with abortion problems as can Release (above).

London Youth Advisory Centre (general counselling), 31 Nottingham Place, London W1. 01-935 1219/ 8870.

Alcoholics Anonymous, 11 Redcliffe Gardens, London SW10 9BH. 01-352 9669 has about 400 local groups.

British Council for the Rehabilitation of the Disabled Tavistock House South, Tavistock Square, London WC1H 9LB. 01-387 4037.

National Association for Mental Health, 39 Queen Anne Street, London W1M 0AJ. 01-935 1272.

British Red Cross Society, 14 Grosvenor Crescent, London SW1X 7EE. 01-235 7131. has many branches which loan commodes, wheelchairs etc., also run holiday homes for the disabled.

Age Concern, 55 Gower Street, London WC1E 6HJ. 01-637 2886 are concerned with old people.

Glossary

denoids: tissue in the
larynx which may become
swollen and give rise to
distorted speech.

mino acids: organic acids
containing nitrogen from
which proteins are built and
which are the basis for life.

naemia: a deficiency of red
ood cells or of haemoglobin
of both.

ntibiotic: a substance
oduced by a mould which
s the power of destroying
cro-organisms. Many are
ed in the treatment of
fectious diseases and some
n be produced synthetically.
e most famous is penicillin.

tery: a vessel which carries
ood away from the heart.

sal metabolic rate—
MR: the metabolic rate of a
ting person.

orhythm: biological
rhythm or cycle of behaviour
oduced by the action of
nute quantities of chemical
ostances; the most
vious biorhythm being
ep.

ood transfusion: the
ocess of injecting blood
m one person into the
od of another.

ecum: part of the large
estine.

lorie: a unit of heat used
express energy levels in the
dy. It is properly called a
ocalorie and is the amount
heat needed to raise the
mperature of 1,000 grams of
ter (1 litre) through one
gree centigrade when that

---

water is pure.

Cancer: a malignant growth
or tumour formed by the
uncontrolled multiplication of
cells which may spread
throughout a tissue causing its
degeneration.

Capillary: a minute blood
vessel, a complex of which
connect an artery with a vein.

Carbohydrate: any one of a
group of substances containing
carbon, hydrogen and oxygen
in the proportion $Cx(H_2O)y$
where x and y can be almost
any number. Starches, sugars
and cellulose are all carbohydrates.

Cell: one unit of protoplasm
and the smallest part of a
living thing, each cell
contains a nucleus which
reproduces by sub-dividing.

Chromosome: a structure in
the nucleus of a cell through
which hereditary characteristics
are passed on by means of
genes.

Circadian rhythm: the daily
24 hour cycle of biorhythms.

Clitoris: the female equivalent
in sexual activity of the male
penis.

Coccyx: the lowest bone of
the vertebral column formed
by the fusion of several
vertebra and being all that
remains of the tail.

Cochlea: the spirally coiled
tube in the inner ear, part of
the organ of hearing.

Colon: the main part of the
large intestine extending from
the caecum to the rectum.

Colour blindness: condition
of sight in which some colours
cannot be appreciated.

Conjunctivitis: inflammation
of the transparent layer
covering the surface of the eye.

Dehydration: a bodily state
brought about by lack of water.

Dermis: a layer of skin
below the epidermis which
contains the roots of hairs,
sweat glands etc.

Diaphragm: a more or less
dome-shaped partition made
of muscle which separates the
chest from the stomach cavity
and allows us to breathe.

Diastolic pressure: the
relaxation of the heart causing
the in-flow of blood.

Digestion: the breakdown of
complex food substances into
simple compounds by the
action of enzymes.

DNA: deoxyribonucleic acid,
the acid composing the
nucleus of the genetic part of
chromosomes.

Energy: capacity for doing
work, derived in the body
from the conversion of heat
which we measure in
calories.

Enzyme: a complex organic
substance, which has the
power to alter the rate of
chemical reactions, important
for the digestion of food.

Epidermis: the outer layer
of skin.

Excretion: the removal of
waste materials from the body
which have been formed during
metabolism.

Faeces: the solid waste
removed from the digestive
system via the anus.

Fats: one of the main groups
of food substances, complex
organic substances which are
insoluble in water.

Gall bladder: a sac for
storing bile between meals.
As soon as food arrives in
the stomach the bile is
secreted.

Gene: the unit of inheritance,
a particular piece of a
chromosome responsible for
the inheritance of
characteristics.

Glucose: a simple form of
sugar which can easily be
converted in the body into
energy.

Haemoglobin: the pigment
found in blood which absorbs
oxygen, it contains iron and

is closely related to chlorophyll. Bright red when oxygenated, bluish-red when deoxygenated.

Haemophilia: a disease occurring in males only, in which blood clotting does not function properly, is transmitted by inheritance.

Hormones: organic substances which act as chemical messengers being carried from one part of the body to another in the blood.

Hypertension: high blood pressure.

Iron: stored in the liver, built into the haemoglobin molecule. Dietary lack causes anaemia.

Jaundice: a disease caused by a liver disorder upsetting bile distribution.

Kidney: the organ which filters liquid waste products and also helps to maintain the correct salt balance.

Leukaemia: cancer-like disease of the blood.

Liver: the largest organ of the body with many functions including the storage of glycogen and the manufacture of bile.

Menstrual cycle: the rhythmic changes in the female reproductive system in which the wall of the uterus is prepared for the implantation of the fertilised egg. If this does not occur, the inner layer of the uterus is ejected, causing menstrual flow.

Metabolism: the sum total of all chemical changes occurring in the body.

Mongolism: a condition of mental and physical retardation related to a chromosome deficiency.

Myopia: short-sightedness—caused when the light rays are focused too far in front of the retina and the object thus appears out of focus.

Nerve: a bundle of nerve fibres rather like the bundle of telephone wires seen down a man-hole, though in miniature.

Nicotinic acid: nicotinamide —Vitamin B_3, found in yeast, meat and fish.

Obesity: fatness.

Organ: a part of the body which forms a functional unit, e.g. kidney, heart, eye.

Oxyhaemoglobin: haemoglobin combined with oxygen, unstable in regions of low oxygen, thus giving up its oxygen where needed.

Pancreas: produces various enzymes which are secreted into the digestive tract, also responsible for secreting insulin into the blood.

Penicillium: a mould from which the antibiotic penicillin is produced, although usually synthesised today.

Penis: organ used to eject urine in the male, and in reproduction to introduce sperm into the female.

Pituitary gland: an important endocrine gland, situated under the brain, which secretes many hormones.

Placenta: attaches the embryo to the uterus of the mother and provides the means of nourishing the embryo.

Plasma: the fluid content of blood in which the blood cells float, plasma can be seen when a blister bursts.

Poliomyelitis: polio—an acute disease caused by a virus resulting in the paralysis of various muscles.

Prostate gland: a gland of the male reproductive system which contributes to the production of semen.

Protein: highly complex organic compound composed of numerous amino acids, the main body-building food substances.

Rectum: the last part of the intestine opening to the exterior at the anus.

Retina: the light-sensitive layer of the eye containing receptor cells known as rods and cones.

Riboflavin: Vitamin B_2 found in yeast, and milk, necessary for a healthy skin condition.

Rickets: a malformation of bones owing to a lack of calcium or Vitamin D or of both.

Roughage: cellulose material which stimulates the bowel to action.

Saliva: fluid containing ptaylin, secreted from the salivary glands as a reflex action resulting from the presence of food in the mouth The thought of food may also stimulate secretions, hence "mouth-watering".

Scurvy: a deficiency disease caused by a lack of Vitamin C

Semi-circular canals: tubes in the inner ear which control balance.

Spinal cord: the central nervous system excluding the brain.

Stroke: rupture of arteries supplying the brain with bloo

Systolic pressure: the contraction of the heart forcir the blood out.

Thiamine: Vitamin B_1, deficiency causes beri-beri.

Thyroid: endocrine gland in the neck region which secrete thyroxin.

Trachea: the windpipe.

Umbilical cord: a stalk joining the placenta to the embryo in the mother throug which nourishment passes.

Uterus: part of the female reproductive system in which the embryo forms.

Vein: a vessel taking deoxygenated blood towards the heart.

Virus: a disease-causing agent which is on the border line between living and non-living. Can only reproduce in a living cell.

ndex

umbers in *italics* indicate
ustrations.

bdomen, 19, 23, 28, 30, 31, 55
cne, 47, 66
denoids, 91
drenal glands, 14, 53, 54, *84*
drenalin, 52, 53, 54, 91
cohol, 31, 32
coholism, 35, 91
lergy, 13, 26
mino acids, 91, 93
mphetamine, 39
naemia, 26, 59, 77, 91, 92
nnular ligament, *83*
ntibodies, 26, 27
ntibiotic, 91
ntihistamine cream, 65
ntiseptic, 46, 64
nus, 49, 92, 93
ppendix, 49, 50, *85*
teries, 22, 23, 24, *25*, 28, 29, 33, 39, 41, 68, *84*, 91
thritis, 18
tificial hip joint, 19
tificial respiration, 62
spirin, 64, 55
las vertebra, 18
ditory nerve, *44*
ricle, *33*
stralian aborigine, 11
straloid type, *11*
stralopithecus, 7, *8*
tomatic nervous system, 34, 34
is vertebra, 18
con, 34, 37

, B$_{12}$ vitamins, 77
cteria, 14
lding, 47, 68
ll and socket joint, *18*
ceps, *83*
nocular vision, 6, 43
rhythm, 12, 15
th, 13, *58*, 59, 81

Blackhead, 47
Bladder, 22, 30, 31, 32, *85*
Blindness, 42
Blind spot, *45*
Blood, 14, 22, 23, 24, 26, 27, 28, 29, 30, 31, 33, 34, 39, 47, 54, 58, 76, 91,
Blood group, 26
Blood pressure, 13, 28, 29
Bloodstream, 12, 15, 19, 26, 32, 48, 49, 52, 53, 54, 55, 57, 58
Blood transfusion, *26*, 91
Blood vessels, 4, 23, 24, 26, 27, 28, *29*, 31, 46, 91
Bone, 16, 18, 19, 20, 43, 50, 59, 60, 61, *68*, 77
Bone cell, 16, *17*
Bone marrow, 26, 27
Bowel cancer, 50
Brachial plexus, *86*
Brachioradial, *83*
Braille, *42*
Brain, 4, 6, 7, 9, 13, 16, 28, 29, 30, 32, 34, 36, 37, 38, 39, 40, 41, 42, 43, 44, 52, 53, 60, 61, 62, 92, 93
Brain cells, 39
Brain tumour, 41
Brain waves, 37
Breast, 55, 61
Breathing, 19, 23, 30, 34, 62, 63, 92
Bronchi, 30
Brochioles, 30
Bronchitis, 30
Burns, 42, 64

Caecum, 49, 91
Caffeine, 39
Calamine lotion, 64
Calcium, 59, 77, 78, 79, 93
Calcium phosphate, 19
Calory, 91, 92
Carotene, 91
Cancer, 27, 81, 91,
Carpals, *82*
Cap, 55
Capillary, 24, 28, 49, 91
Carbohydrate, 76, 91
Carbon dioxide, 28, 30, 91
Cardiovascular disease, 76
Cartilage, 16, 18, 19, 61
Caucasoids, *10*
Cauda equina, *86*
Cells, 5, *5*, 14, 16, *17*, 19, 27, 31, 57, 58, 60, 61, 91

Cerebellum, *86*
Cerebrum, *86*,
Cervix, 55, 56, 57, 59
Chair sits, *71*
Chloride, 77
Chlorophyll, 92
Cholesterol, 33, 68, 76
Chromosomes, 58, 91, 92
Cilia, 30
Circadian rhythm, 12, 14, 15
Circulation, 23, 28, 33, 34, 59, 61, 68
Cirrhotic, 31
Clavicle, *82*
Clitoris, 56, 91
Clotting, 24, 26, 77, 91, 92
Coccyx, *82*, 91
Cochlea, *44*, 91
Cold, 62
Colon, 49, 50, *85*, 91
Colour blindness, 73, 91
Conception, 55, 57
Condom, 55
Congoid group, 11
Conjunctivitis, 91
Connective tissues, 5
Constipation, 50, 65
Contortionist, *16*
Contraceptives, 55
Copper, 77
Cornea, *45*, 68
Corpus spongiosum, *56*
Cramp, 23
Cranium, *82*,
Cro-magnon man, *9*
Cuticles, 67
Cystitis, 31

Dandruff, 68
Darwin, Charles, 6
Deafness, 43
Death, 13, 27, 29, 51, 54, 60, 81
Dehydration, 91
Delivery, 58, 59
Dental floss, 67
Deltoid, *83*
Dentine, 67
Deodorant, 52
Deoxyribonucleic acid (DNA) 91
Depression, 39
Dermis, 46, 91
Diabetes, 54
Diaphragm, 30, 91
Diarrhoea, 48, 50, 65

Diastolic blood pressure, 13
91
Diet, 50, 51, 65, 68, 71, 76, 77
Digestion, 28, 34, 48, 49, 52,
65, 76, 91
Digestive system, 42, 48, 49,
50, 54, 77, 81, 92
Diptheria, 35
Disinfectant, 64
Diuretic drug, 15
Dorsal ecercise, 70
Drugs, 14
Duodenum, 49,

Ear, 42, 93
Ear canal, 44
Ear-drum, 43, 44, 61
Eczma, 47
Egg, 57, 58, 92
Electrodes, 38
Electroencephalogram, 38
Electro-encephalograph, 37, 38
Embryo, 4, 57, 58, 93
Emotions, 74, 75
Encephalitis, 41
Endocrine glands, 52, 53,
84, 93
Endometrium, 57
Energy, 78, 79, 91
Enzymes, 48, 49, 51, 91
Epidermal cells, 47
Epilepsy, 14, 41
Eskimos, 10
Ethnoid palate, 45
European type, 10
Eustachian tube, 44
Escher, Maurits, 72
Excretion, 13, 32, 34, 91
Exercises, 22, 68, 70, 71
Expiratory peak flow, 13
Extensor carpi ulnaris, 83
Eye, 7, 43, 57, 68, 72, 92

Faeces, 48, 49, 50, 91
Fallopian tubes, 57, 58
False teeth, 62
Fat, 76, 91
Feet, 44, 68
Femur, 82
Fertilisation, 58
Fibrogen, 26
Fibula, 82
Fingernails, 4, 67
First aid, 62
Florida, 15
Fluoride, 67, 77

Foetus, 58, 59
Folic acid, 77
Follicle, 47, 67
Foreplay, 56
Foreskin, 56
Food, 4, 23, 24, 43, 48, 49, 50,
51, 62, 76, 78, 92
Frontal lobe, 86

Gage, Phineas, 37
Gall bladder, 31, 85, 91
Ganglion, 35, 36, 86
Gastric ulcers, 54
Gastrocnemeus, 83
Genes, 27, 58, 91, 91
Glands, 26, 52, 58, 91
Glans, 56
Glucose, 22, 24, 31, 54, 91
Gluteus maximus, 83
Glycogen, 2, 92
Goitre, 54, 77, 92
Gout, 51
Granulocytes, 26
Grasp reflex, 35
Gustatory cell, 45
Gut, 32, 50, 51, 53, 60

Haemoglobin, 24, 26, 77, 91,
91
Haemophilia, 27, 92
Haemorrhage, 27
Haemorrhoids, 50, 65
Hair, 10, 11, 46, 47, 52, 58,
61, 67, 68, 91
Half squats, 70,
Hamstrings, 83
Hangover, 65
Hay-fever, 26
Headache, 12, 41, 62, 65
Hearing, 38, 40, 43
Hearing aid, 43
Heart, 5, 19, 22, 24, 28, 30,
32, 33, 52, 53, 59, 81, 85,
91, 93
Hearbeat, 22
Heartburn, 50, 65
Heart rate, 13
Heart valves, 30
Hinge joints, 18
Hip, 18, 19
Homo erectus, 7, 8, 9
Homo habilis, 7
Homo sapiens, 7, 8
Hormones, 12, 14, 15, 22, 31,
34, 47, 49, 53, 54, 55, 91,
92

Humerus, 82
Hydrochloric acid, 49
Hypertension, 28, 29

Indigestion, 50, 54
Indonesia, 7
Infection, 12, 24
Insomnia, 12
Insulin, 49, 54, 93
Intestines, 22, 31, 32, 34, 48,
49, 51, 54, 60, 85, 91
Intra Uterine Device (IUD), 5!
Involuntary muscle, 20, 22
Iodine, 54, 77, 92
Iris, 45
Iron, 26, 59, 77, 78, 79, 92
Iron deficiency, 47

Jaundice, 92
Java man, 9
Jet-lag, 12
Joints, 16, 18, 19, 20, 51, 61,
68
Jumps, 71

Keratin, 47
Kidney, 24, 28, 29, 31, 32, 51
53, 85, 92, 93
Kilocalories, 78, 91
Knee joint, 18

Labour, 59
Lactic acid, 22, 23
Lake Rudolf, 6, 7
Laxatives, 65
Leakey, Richard, 6
Leg lifts, 71
Lens, 45
Leukemia, 27
Life expectancy, 81
Ligament, 16, 18
Limbs, 6, 20, 22, 23, 28, 38,
Lingual nerve, 45
Lips, 11, 44
Liver, 31, 32, 49, 51, 85, 92
Longevity, 60
LSD, 39
Lumbo-sacral plexus, 86
Lunatic, 14
Lung, 19, 28, 29, 30, 32, 33,
53, 54, 62, 85
Lung cancer, 30
Lymph, 24, 84
Lymph nodes, 26
Lymphocytes, 26

Madness, 14
Magnesium, 77
Malnutrition, 47
Mandible, 82
Manic depression, 15
Marceau, Marcel, *22*
Masai tribe, 50
Median nerve, *86*
Melancholy, 15
Melanesian, 11
Melanin pigment, 46
Membranes, 18, 41
Meningitis, 41
Menopause, 47, 61
Menstruation, 15
Menstrual cycle, 14, 15, 92
Mental disturbance, 15
Mental hospitals, 15
Metabolism, 92
Metatarsals, *82*
Migrane, 41
Mongolism, 92
Mongoloids, *10*
Morning sickness, 59
Mouth, 30, 43, 49, 52, 62, 63, 91
Mucus, 30, 43, 49, 51, 57
Muscle, 16, *20*, 22, 23, 30, 36, 42, 43, 54, 61, 68, 70, 92,
Muscle tone, 23, 48
Multiple sclerosis, 34
Myelin sheath, 34, 35
Myopia, 92

Nails, 6, 47, *67*
Neanderthal man, 7, *9*
Negroid group, *11*
Nerve, 34, 35, 36, 37, 40, *44*, *45*, 92
Nerve cells, 34, 38, 60
Nerve endings, 42
Nervous system, 20, 22, 34, 35, 52, 53, 60, *86*
Neuralgia, 35
Neuron, 34, 35, 36, 37, 38
Neurosurgeon, 37
Neuro-transmitter, 38, 39
Niacin, 77, 79
Nicotinic acid, 77, 92
Nutrients, 12, 24, 31, 39, 49, 57, 58, 76, 77, 78

Obesity, 81, 92
Obturator nerve, *86*
Oesophagus, 49, 50
Oldurai Gorge, 7

Olfactory bulb, *45*
Olfactory membrane, *45*
Olfactory receptors, 43
Optic nerve, *45*
Oral body remperature, 13
Organ, 4, *5*, 14, 19, 23, 24, 28, 31, 32, 34, 46, 49, 53, 54, 55, 56, 57, 58, 60, 61, 92
Organism, 14, 24
Orgasm, 56
Ovaries, 32, 55, 57, 58, 61
Oviducts, 58
Oxygen, 23, 24, 26, 28, 30, 39, 54, 59, 77, 91
Oxy-haemoglobin, 24, 92

Pain, 13, 14, 34, 36, 42
Pain-killers, 14
Palate, *45*
Pancreas, 31, *49*, 54, *84*, 92
Papillae, *45*
Paralysis, 29
Parasite, 81
Patella, *82*
Pectoralis major, *83*
Pekin man, *9*
Pellagra, 77
Pelvis, 19, 55, *82*
Penicillium, 93
Penis, 31, 55, *56*, 58, 91, 92
Period, 57
Peristalsis, 22, 49,
Peristalstic movement, 34
Perspiration, 23, 46
Phalanges, *82*
Pharynx, 91
Pheromenes, 15
Phosphorus, 77
Photomicrograph, 16, *17*
Pill, 55
Pituitary gland, 53, *84*, 92
Pivot joint, *18*
Placenta, 57, 58, 59, 92
Plaque, 66, 67
Plasma, 13, 24, 26, 31
Platelets, 24, 26
Poliomyelitis, 92
Potassium, 77, 92
Pregnancy, 6, 47, 55, 59, 77
Premenstrual tension, 15
Press-ups, *70*, 71
Proconsul, *8*
Prostrate gland, 31, *56*, 92
Protoplasm, 91

Protein, 13, 24, 48, 49, 76, 78, 79, 91, 92
Ptyalin, 49
Pupil, *45*
Pyloric sphincter, *49*

Radial nerve, *86*
Radius, *82*
Receptors, 23, 36, 42, *45*, 46
Rectum, 49, *85*, 91, 92
Rectus femoris, *83*
Red blood cells, 24, 26, 27, 28, 30, 31, 77, 91
Reflex arc, 36
Reproduction, 34, 55, 58
Resilient lens, 43
Respiration, 34
Retina, *45*, 92, 92
Rhesus factor, 27
Rheumatic illness, 68
Rh-negative, 27
Rhodesia man, *9*
Rh-positive, 27
Rib, 19, 30, 32, *82*
Rib-cage, 30
Riboflavin, 77, 79, 92
Rickets, *50*, 93

Sacrum, *82*
Saddle joints, *18*
Sciatic nerve, *86*
Scurvey, 93
St. Martin, Alexis, 28
Saliva, 43, 49, 62, 67, 92
Salivary glands, 52
Salt tablets, 23
Sartorius, *83*
Scalp, 67, 68
Scapula, *82*
Scrotum, *56*
Sebaceous glands, 46, 47, 52, 67
Sebum, 46, 47
Secretory neuron, 36
Semen, 56, 93
Semi-circular canals, *44*, 92
Seminal vesicles, 56
Senility, 39, 60, 61, 71
Sense organs, 41, 44
Sensory vein, *44*
Sexual intercourse, 55, *56*, 58
Shaving, 47
Sheath, 55
Shingles, 35
Short-sightedness, 43
Side-bending, *70*

Sight, 40, 43
Sit-ups, 70
Skeleton, 4, 7, 8, 16, 17, 77,
Skin, 4, 13, 20, 36, 42, 46,
   47, 52, 53, 61, 64, 66, 68
Skin cell, 46
Skin nerve, 44
Skull, 16, 18. 20, 43, 60
Sleeps, 12, 22, 39
Slipped disc, 68
Smell, 6, 42, 43
Sodium, 77
Solo man, 9
Sound waves, 43
Speech, 40
Sperm, 55, 56, 57, 58
Sphincter, 49
Spinal Column, 16
Spinal cord, 16, 34, 35, 36,
   86, 93
Spinal nerve, 34
Spine, 18, 23, 30, 35, 61
Spleen, 26, 85,
Splinter, 64, 65
Spot running, 70
Sprain, 42
Starches, 49, 76, 91
Sternum, 82
Stomach, 28, 32, 48, 49, 50,
   61, 70, 85, 91, 92
Stomach wall, 49
Stroke, 29
Sterno-cleido mastoid, 83
Substances, 38
Sunburn, 64, 66

Sweat, 46, 47, 52
Sympathetic outflow, 86
Syphilis, 41,
Systolic blood pressure, 13

Tartar, 67
Tarus, 82
Taste, 42, 43, 61
Taste bud, 45
Teeth, 6, 49, 61, 66, 67, 77
Temporal lobe, 86
Tendon, 20, 36, 42
Tensor fascia lata, 83
Testicles, 32, 56, 58, 84
Thiamine, 77, 92
Thigh bone, 19
Three-bone lever, 44
Thrombocytes, 26
Thumb, 18
Thymus, 26
Thyroid gland, 54, 84, 92, 93
Thyroxin, 91, 92, 92
Tibia, 82
Tibialis anticus, 83
Tissue, 4, 5, 16, 19, 20, 22,
   24, 28, 37, 39, 46, 47, 48,
   61, 66, 76, 77, 91
Toenails, 4
Toes, 18
Tongue, 43, 62
Touch, 42, 44
Toxin, 50
Trachea, 30, 85, 92
Trapezius, 83
Triceps, 83

Trunk, 32
Trunk-raising, 71
Tumour, 91

Ultra-violet radiation, 46, 64
Umbilical cord, 59, 92
Ureters, 31
Urethra, 31, 56
Uric acid, 51
Urination, 31, 58
Urine, 13, 93
Uterus, 55, 57, 58, 59, 92,
   92

Vagina, 55, 58, 59
Varicose veins, 28
Vastas medialis, 83
Vein, 28, 84, 91, 92
Ventricles, 33
Vertebra, 16, 18, 82, 91
Vertebrate, 16
Victoria, Queen of England, 27
Villi, 49
Virus, 34, 92
Vitamins, 46, 76, 79, 91
Vitamin deficiency, 50
Vitreous humour, 45
Voluntary muscle, 20, 22, 23
Vomit, 62
Vulva, 59

Weight. 13, 71, 87
White blood cells, 26, 27, 60
Womb, 55, 57, 59

Credits

Artists
Allard Design Group Ltd.
Ron Hayward Art Group
Oxford Illustrators
Tony Mould
Tony Payne
QED
Sidney Woods

Photographs
Al Heath International: 16
St. Bartholomew's Hospital:
   Contents, 50
British Museum: Contents, 51
British Museum (Natural
   History): 7
Camera Press: 30

Bob Campbell: 6
R. J. Chilton: 31
Colorsport: Contents
Gene Cox: 17
Daily Telegraph: 69
Glyn Davies: 26
Ebury Press: 41
Escher Foundation/
   Gemeetemuseum
   The Hague: 72
Ronald Grant: 52
Health Education Council: 55
"The Insane in Foreign
   Countries", Letchworth: 14
"Tests for Colour Blindness',
   S. Ishihara: 73
Le Roye: 21
Peggy Leder: 22, 23

Marshall Cavendish Ltd: 35
Mansell Collection, London: 27
Novosti Press Agency: 60
Popperfoto: 47
Pictorial Press Ltd: 59
Radio Times Hulton Picture
   Library: Contents, 58
Roche: 38
Royal College of Surgeons:
   Contents, 19
Syndication International Ltd.
   London: 42, 54
John Watney Photo Library: 28
   29

Cover
Design: Barry Kemp
Photograph: Paul Forrester